MEASURING SOCIETY

ASA-CRC Series on
**STATISTICAL REASONING IN SCIENCE AND
SOCIETY**

SERIES EDITORS

Nicholas Fisher, University of Sydney, Australia
Nicholas Horton, Amherst College, MA, USA
Deborah Nolan, University of California, Berkeley, USA
Regina Nuzzo, Gallaudet University, Washington, DC, USA
David J Spiegelhalter, University of Cambridge, UK

PUBLISHED TITLES

Errors, Blunders, and Lies: How to Tell the Difference
David S. Salsburg

Visualizing Baseball
Jim Albert

Data Visualization: Charts, Maps and Interactive Graphics
Robert Grant

Improving Your NCAA® Bracket with Statistics
Tom Adams

Statistics and Health Care Fraud: How to Save Billions
Tahir Ekin

Measuring Crime: Behind the Statistics
Sharon Lohr

Measuring Society
Chaitra H. Nagaraja

For more information about this series, please visit:
https://www.crcpress.com/go/asacrc

MEASURING SOCIETY

CHAITRA H. NAGARAJA

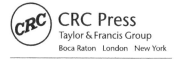

CRC Press
Taylor & Francis Group
Boca Raton   London   New York

CRC Press is an imprint of the
Taylor & Francis Group, an **informa** business

A CHAPMAN & HALL BOOK

CRC Press
Taylor & Francis Group
6000 Broken Sound Parkway NW, Suite 300
Boca Raton, FL 33487-2742

© 2020 by Taylor & Francis Group, LLC
CRC Press is an imprint of Taylor & Francis Group, an Informa business

No claim to original U.S. Government works

International Standard Book Number-13: 978-1-138-03598-0 (Paperback)
International Standard Book Number-13: 978-0-367-27517-4 (Hardback)

Library of Congress Cataloging-in-Publication Data

Names: Nagaraja, Chaitra H., author.
Title: Measuring society / Chaitra H. Nagaraja.
Description: Boca Raton : CRC Press, Taylor & Francis Group, 2019. | Includes
bibliographical references and index.
Identifiers: LCCN 2019011127| ISBN 9781138035980 (pbk. : alk. paper) | ISBN
9780367275174 (hardback : alk. paper)
Subjects: LCSH: Mathematics--Popular works. | Statistics--Popular works. |
Economics--Mathematical models.
Classification: LCC QA93 .N3255 2019 | DDC 306.301/51--dc23
LC record available at https://lccn.loc.gov/2019011127

Visit the Taylor & Francis Web site at
http://www.taylorandfrancis.com

and the CRC Press Web site at
http://www.crcpress.com

To LB

There may be [a] wide difference of opinion as to the significance of a very unequal distribution of wealth, but there can be no doubt as to the importance of knowing whether the present distribution is becoming more or less unequal.

M.O. Lorenz, 1905

Contents

Preface   xi

CHAPTER   1 ▪ Introduction   1

CHAPTER   2 ▪ Jobs   5

CHAPTER   3 ▪ Inequality   25

CHAPTER   4 ▪ Housing   51

CHAPTER   5 ▪ Prices   71

CHAPTER   6 ▪ Poverty   97

CHAPTER   7 ▪ Deprivation   127

CHAPTER   8 ▪ Postscript   151

Glossary   155

Bibliography   163

Index   173

Preface

While watching the news during the 2016 U.S. presidential election, I, like many others, became exasperated. It was frustrating to see countless official statistics, like unemployment and poverty rates, bandied about with little thought as to what they were measuring and why. This book is a result of that frustration.

I first became interested in official statistics through my research with Lawrence D. Brown, my marvelous Ph.D. advisor. Larry was enthusiastic about this project, though, sadly, he passed away before its completion. This book is dedicated to him.

Royalty checks accrue to the author, but every book is inevitably the sum of many people's efforts. I am grateful to the editors of the ASA-CRC Series on Statistical Reasoning in Science and Society—Nicholas Fisher, Nicholas Horton, Deborah Nolan, Regina Nuzzo, and David Spiegelhalter—for taking a chance on a person writing her first book. I'm also extremely grateful to the reviewers—David Giles from the University of Victoria, William Nicholson from Cornell University, and Mark Scanlan from Stephen F. Austin State University—who offered their time and expertise to provide helpful feedback. (Obviously, any errors are my own.)

A special thanks to my sister, Smitha, and my husband, Kartik. Both read and commented extensively on my drafts. Kartik even supplemented these comments with many ploughman's lunches. I also couldn't have finished this book without the encouragement of my parents, H.N. and Jyothi, and my in-laws, Meena and Chico.

I'd like to acknowledge: Aaron Polhamus and Valuation Technology Inc. (ValuTech) for allowing me to use their data for the housing chapter; Stephen Ornes for helping to rethink my chapter on inequality measures; Fr. Vincent DeCola and Karina Hogan from Fordham University for their help on the story of Abraham and Lot; Trudi Renwick and Brian Glassman from the U.S. Census Bureau along with Thesia Garner from the Bureau of Labor Statistics for their assistance with the Supplemental Poverty Measure threshold calculations; and Jonathan Church from the Bureau of Labor Statistics for his help with rebasing inflation measures. Thanks as well to Sherry Thomas, Michele Dimont, Shashi Kumar, and others at CRC Press for their assistance during production.

Given the lengthy list of references, it goes without saying that libraries are awesome. This book would have been devoid of fun facts without the resources at the Fordham University Libraries, the New York Public Library, the Upper Arlington Public Library, and many digital archives, including the National Agricultural Library in Bethesda, Maryland, the National Archives and Records Administration, and the HathiTrust Digital Library.

A final and heartfelt thank you goes to my cheery and wise editor, John Kimmel, who kept me on track. Yay, we're done!

Chaitra H. Nagaraja
New York

CHAPTER 1

Introduction

O UR WORLD swirls with percentages, ratios, and graphs. Unfortunately, the numbers that we encounter in real life—like unemployment and inflation—are usually stated but left unexplained.

These numbers are examples of official statistics. They are reported to cause alarm, insinuate a sleight of hand by the government, or brag about "results." No one really bothers to clarify what these weighty terms actually mean. Regrettably, this severely limits our ability to assess claims made in the news or by our politicians.

While this book's title implies it is rooted in statistics, its content emphasizes that history is important too. This is because official measures are an inseparable mix of politics and statistics.

Interpreting what official statistics can and cannot tell us is crucial. Understanding *why* they were poked and prodded into being measured that way is just as significant, if not more so.

To measure a human-designed society requires human-designed measures, with all attendant foibles folded into them. Consequently, thinking about these measures requires an apparatus more akin to the investigative journalist's "Who? What? Why? Where? When? How?" inventory than a physicist's scale and ruler. Here are some things we will consider:

1. **What will this measure be used for?** The purpose of a measure will likely vary over time. Therefore, the measure itself must be updated to reflect that shift in purpose.

2. **What is being measured? Is it practical?** If you want to survey lawyers about their salaries, an easy way would be to wander the streets foraging for attorneys. However, who

you find depends on the time of day, if the area is commercial or residential, and even where in the country you are. All of these factors make it unlikely you can assume that the people you find are representative of lawyers in the city, let alone in the country. And so, you're left holding some bits of data and no way to draw a general conclusion about lawyers.

3. **Is it possible to collect information about this topic?** Often the answer to this is a resounding no. For instance, if you want to measure poverty, you can't simply go around asking people if they are poor. That word will mean different things to different people. Instead, you need to define the abstract concept of what it means to be poor; this is where formulas become useful. The data you collect will be determined by that very specific definition.

4. **Is the information you are collecting actually measuring what you think you are measuring?** You may call a formula a poverty rate, but it's really just shorthand for "fraction of people who live in households earning below a set amount calculated using a method from the 1960s." Or maybe it's shorthand for "fraction of people who feel like they are poor" or even the "fraction of people who can't afford to own a dog." These are all different things, some more related to poverty than others. You need to be able to justify that what you are measuring—your formula—is actually what you want to learn about. For example, if you want to learn about poverty, perhaps looking at dog ownership isn't the best plan. Sure, broke people can't afford pets, but is this really telling you what you want to know?

5. **How are you collecting this data?** Once you have a formula, you must have a plan so people can actually go out and gather some data. That plan has to allow for two things. First, you should be able to use your formula with the data collected. This seems obvious, but implementing a study is difficult. Second, in order for a measure to have meaning beyond describing the people who participated in the study, the data must be collected in accordance with statistical principles. This is also tough to do in practice.

6. **Is there a correct answer?** When it comes to statistics about people and their lives, the answer to this question is

either "definitely not" or "in theory, yes." Questions 3 and 4 refer to how well the formula (i.e., measure) matches the concept. Question 5 looks at how well we can implement the formula in practice. We can apply the, "Is there a correct answer?" question to both. For the former, the answer is "definitely not" because the formula is simply one way of looking at a concept. For the latter, however, the answer is "in theory, yes." Better data collection techniques and surveying more people (or objects) can get our estimates closer to what the formulas intend.

7. **Will you be calculating this statistic once or regularly?** This question determines whether you care enough about the measure to see how it changes across months or years. That, in turn, affects how much time and money you are willing to spend on this exercise now and in the future.

8. **Do you care about this measure across different geographical areas?** Depending on the purpose of a statistic, you might want to calculate one number for the entire country or one for each state, county, or school district. In the end, what you decide to do again depends on how much time/money/energy you have, regardless of your goals.

Measures about six topics are discussed in this book: jobs, inequality, house prices, prices for goods and services, poverty, and deprivation. Each of these is debated in politics, used to make government policy, and contributes to an understanding of the society in which we live. Versions of these statistics (official and unofficial) float around the news. A few are even used to describe shifts in business cycles (you may have heard of leading and lagging economic indicators).

On an individual level, these measures are formal versions of ways we already use to form an understanding of the society around us: We need a job, a place to live, and food to eat. We also compare ourselves with others and these measures inevitably reflect that tendency.

Now for some administrative stuff before we begin. This is a nearly formula-free book; there is only one bona fide formula in here. If needed, a glossary of terms and data sources can be found at the end. Finally, each chapter concludes with a few selections if you want to continue reading about a particular topic. We start here with a pair of articles, one written by a user of statistics, the other by a producer.

FURTHER READING

"Tim Harford's guide to statistics in a misleading age," by Tim Harford. *Financial Times*, February 8, 2018.

Harford offers people—statisticians and non-statisticians alike—a short list about what to keep in mind when encountering a statistic. He starts with "observe your feelings." This is practical advice as many facts and figures that catch our eye are on subjects about which we feel most strongly. It also reminds us those statistics are often created by people who are keen on that subject too.

"Living with symbols," by Arthur M. Ross. *The American Statistician*, 1966.

When he wrote this article, Ross was Commissioner of the Bureau of Labor Statistics at the U.S. Department of Labor. This is the federal agency that publishes, among other things, statistics on unemployment and inflation. With a tongue-in-cheek tone, he talks about the unavoidably ambiguous nature of measuring all things social and economic.

CHAPTER 2

Jobs

O N OCTOBER 24ᵀᴴ, 1929, the stock market crashed. Black Thursday slid into Black Tuesday when, on the 29ᵗʰ, the market crashed again. Panic spread.

President Herbert Hoover was not entirely convinced that things were so bad. His pet theory was that this was a blip in the economy and that soon—very soon—things would settle down and simply go back to normal.

To prove it, his administration began collecting information on unemployment. Hoover was certain this new data would silence his adversaries. At the end of only a single week, seeing a promising twitch in the statistics, he grandiosely declared his theory correct.[88]

Unfortunately for Hoover, things failed to improve. The market crashes were omens for the Great Depression. Hoover's inability to square his theory with the ground realities ultimately meant he lost the next election to Franklin D. Roosevelt in 1932.

Now, every month, the Bureau of Labor Statistics (BLS), the second largest federal statistical agency in the U.S., publishes the stiffly named "The Employment Situation." It contains lots of statistics including the number of jobs created, the labor force participation rate, and the unemployment rate. It's used to describe the state of the economy. Markets move on the release of this information; political fortunes hinge on it.

The third statistic in the list above, the unemployment rate, is considered a key economic indicator. As firms lay off workers only if times are already bad, the unemployment rate is regarded as a lagging indicator. It reflects changes in the economy that are already occurring.

Provided you know what people do for a living, calculating the unemployment rate does not appear, at first glance, to be onerous. Basically, we have to know how many people there are and count how many of them are unemployed. Once we know those two numbers, we just divide them. (This is called a ratio statistic because we need to determine both parts of the fraction.)

Let's start with who counts as unemployed. For example, say Ezra just moved to Ohio and is currently looking for a nursing job. Is he unemployed? Clearly, yes. How about Claire who just quit her job at a law firm to start a new one next month? She is technically not working today, but she doesn't fit our mental picture of an unemployed person. Finally, what about Milo who is working part-time at a university but hopes to land a more permanent position? How should we count people like Milo who feel they are underemployed?

Suddenly we find ourselves bogged down by lots of details. Perhaps things will be simpler if we switch to counting the total number of people. We can start by restricting our tally to people who are adults, or close to adulthood. In modern times, we aren't expecting ten-year-old Ottos and Ethels to be toiling away in dank coal mines or clanking factories. People in school full-time should probably be left out as well since they are otherwise occupied. Possibly retired people too. As we pare down this list, we are slowly deciding who in the population should be part of the "labor force."

WHO COUNTS?

It's a steamy day in 1790. You've been galloping around town on your horse. You arrive at a house and knock on the door. It opens and you cautiously peer inside. Quill at the ready, you introduce yourself and begin tallying and cataloging the residents. This is your job as an enumerator for the first U.S. census: counting who lives where and (presumably) with great care.

A census is required every ten years by the U.S. Constitution and so, is called the decennial census ("dec"=10). The goal is to literally count every person who lives in the country (not just citizens). This count is then used to determine how many representatives each state sends to Congress, a process called apportionment. (Enumerators were used extensively until 1960, the first year when all census forms were mailed to homes. That said, enumerators still picked up the completed forms from each household that year.[30])

The first census, however, had two extra objectives. First, the population count could be redeployed to "fairly" distribute expenses from the Revolutionary War against the British. It also contained an embryonic count of a specific type of labor force: males who were free, white, and at least sixteen years old. That is, males who were eligible to serve in a fledgling military.[163]

In 1790, there were around 813,000 such males out of a population of just over 3.9 million free and enslaved people.[117] (Age was deemed irrelevant for women, slaves, and non-white free people even though many worked and obviously slaves worked without pay.)

Many government officials felt this number was unexpectedly low because it didn't square with previous population estimates. They even suspected that families pretended to contain fewer people when the enumerator came knocking to avoid being taxed. In the end, the count was accurate; rather, it was the colonial-era population estimates which were too high.[163]

By 1800, many people were pushing for additional questions to be added to the census. They hoped the extra information would help the government pass better laws. For example, the fourth census in 1820 included the first questions about employment, classifying workers as in agriculture, commerce, or manufacturing.[163]

As the years progressed, the instructions to enumerators became increasingly elaborate. The 1870 enumerators were issued a stern warning: "The inquiry, 'Profession, occupation, or trade,' is one of the most important questions of this schedule. Make a study of it." The government wanted them to be specific: "Instead of saying 'packers,' indicate whether you mean 'pork packers' or 'crockery packers,' or 'mule packers.'" They even insisted on them doing some detective work if the resident was unhelpful.[76]

By the time the 1890 census rolled around, enumerators were charged with distinguishing veterinary surgeons from the usual kind; chemists from metallurgists; actors from showmen. Even hucksters and peddlers would now be categorized based on their wares. And as the Industrial Revolution swept through, new jobs such as railroad officials or telegraph office messenger boys were added to the list of occupations.[76]

All of these shifting and burgeoning categories were attempts to measure the absurd concept known as the "gainful worker." The technical definition of a gainful worker was someone who had a paid profession they usually did. It didn't matter if they were doing something else at the moment or hadn't done that "usual" job in many years. This definition lumbered along until the Great Depression when, amidst staggering unemployment, reporting something you usually did was a demonstrably silly exercise.[16]

And so, the 1940 census switched gears. From gainful workers, people began talking about the "labor force." This change in terminology was accompanied by a clearer query: Were you working or looking for work last week? If you were giving piano lessons this week, even if you were trained to be an engineer, then you would be recorded as a music teacher. If you were looking for a new job this week even though you were a cashier last week, you would be listed as seeking work. In both cases, you would be regarded as part of the labor force. This was an easier question to answer.[16]

Eventually, a new statistic materialized: the labor force participation rate. This is the ratio of people in the labor force divided by everyone. (It is then multiplied by 100 to convert the fraction into a percentage.)

We don't want "everyone" to be literally everyone. For instance, children probably should be excluded. Specifically, "everyone" is defined as those who are sixteen or older, not in the military, and not institutionalized (e.g., nursing homes, prisons). This is the group of people who are deemed eligible to work in a (civilian) job. Those who do have a civilian job or have been looking for one in the past four weeks are called the "labor force."

The labor force participation rate, then, indicates what percent of "everyone" is working or available to work. It is computed monthly from Current Population Survey (CPS) data. This survey is currently administered by the Census Bureau, the largest federal statistical agency, on behalf of BLS (more on this later).

The graphs in Figure 2.1 show how this rate has changed since 1948.[19] (The graphs in this figure are examples of time series data because time (day, month, year, etc.) is on the horizontal axis of the graph.)

Figure 2.1A displays two versions of the labor force participation rate. The black, spiky line is the original statistic. With this version of the measure, it can be difficult to interpret changes from one month to the next. A shift could have occurred because there was an underlying change in the economy. Alternatively, it could be because it's June and high school students are getting summer jobs at the pool, or it's November and shops are hiring temporary workers to accommodate the Christmas rush.

A statistical technique called seasonal adjustment removes the second type of fluctuation so we can focus on fundamental shifts to

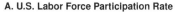

A. U.S. Labor Force Participation Rate

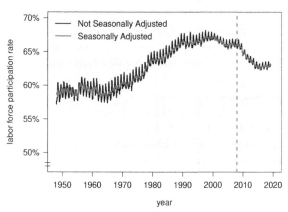

**B. U.S. Labor Force Participation Rate
(Seasonally Adjusted)**

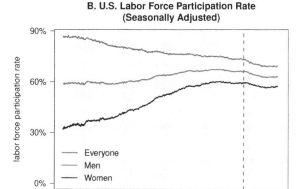

Figure 2.1 Plot A compares the choppier not seasonally adjusted monthly labor force participation rate (black) with the smoother seasonally adjusted one (blue). Plot B shows the same seasonally adjusted monthly rate (again in blue) along with the rate for men (gray) and women (black) separately. The blue lines in both plots are the same; however, the vertical axis scales don't match, which is why they appear different in the graphs. The vertical line at December 2007 marks the start of the Great Recession. (Sources: Current Population Survey; National Bureau of Economic Research.)

the labor force. It results in the smoother blue line in Figure 2.1A, which represents the *seasonally adjusted* labor force participation rate.

In Figure 2.1B, the blue line again represents the seasonally adjusted labor force participation rate. (It's the exact same blue line as in the first plot, but the two plots have different vertical axis scales making it look like the lines are not the same.)

This rate has hovered between 60% and 65% since the late 1940s. There was a dip during the Great Recession after the housing bubble burst in 2007 (dotted line), but it is slight if we take a longer-term perspective.[108] (That said, even small reductions in the labor force participation rate can represent a large number of individuals.)

The roughly 40% of people who are not in the labor force include housewives and househusbands, students, and retirees who aren't in nursing homes. It also includes people who would like a job but have given up looking for one (more on this later).

World War II brought many women into the workforce and plenty of them decided to stay once the war was over, permanently altering the workplace. We can see this trend from the other two lines in Figure 2.1B. Men are shown in gray and women in black. The rate of women in the labor force has steadily increased from around 30% to nearly double that in only 70 years. In fact, rates for men and women appear to be converging and will possibly match each other eventually.

When we group people who have a job and people who are looking for a job together, we have deferred the problem of what counts as a job. We turn to that next by looking at unemployment, a more hotly debated statistic.

BUREAUCRATS ABOUND

After experimenting with various questions about employment, queries about *un*employment were added to the decennial census in 1880. The first results on this topic were published for the 1890 census when occupational data was analyzed from every conceivable angle filling nearly a hundred pages with tables. One of those angles was race.

The 1890 census tables meticulously split whites into three categories: white with American parents, white with foreign parents, and white but foreign born. Everyone else was under the "colored" category with those of "Negro descent" counted as a subset.[59]

This example shows how choosing what data to collect and how to display it reflects the issues and prejudices of the day. The 1800s brought with them a lot of tension regarding immigration. In the middle of the century, many Irish escaped the potato famine by moving to the U.S., giving rise to anti-Irish sentiments, among other ethnic groups. Federal immigration policy was beginning to be codified, starting with the 1875 Page Act which was expanded in 1882 with the Chinese Exclusion Act.[51,52,165]

In subsequent censuses, the questions regarding unemployment changed substantially (including those about race). The minimum age drifted from 10 to 16 years. Unmarried daughters who helped around the home were reclassified as doing "housework—without pay" as opposed to having no occupation at all.[76] All of these changes, large and small, made it difficult to compare unemployment rates from one census to the next.

Nowadays, the U.S. uses a consistent definition of unemployment and the labor force. Furthermore, it gathers this type of data frequently using a set data collection procedure. Getting to this stage shadowed the rising concern about the vast fortunes made in the Gilded Age while laborers worked under dire conditions in factories and mines. These apprehensions induced many people from workers to government officials to act.

We start with Ethelbert Stewart who began his professional life as a lowly worker at the Decatur Coffin Company in Illinois. After being disgusted with how people were treated at his factory, he began writing about it, hoping to improve conditions for workers everywhere. Eventually, he became the head of the Bureau of Labor Statistics (BLS) in 1921 where he made his mark by helping to define and estimate unemployment.[88]

In the early 1920s, President Warren G. Harding, through then Secretary of Commerce (and later president) Herbert Hoover, organized a conference on unemployment. Everyone came away realizing that no one had a clue what the actual unemployment rate was. And so, the American Statistical Association set up the Committee on Governmental Labor Statistics to assist with wording the questions about joblessness for the 1930 census.[28]

By 1937, Roosevelt had unseated Hoover as president. Frances Perkins, the first female U.S. cabinet member, chose Isador Lubin to replace the retiring Stewart as the head of BLS because he would, "remember that statistics were not numbers but people coping or failing to cope with the buffetings of life."[88] Lubin helped make the shift from "gainful worker" to "labor force" in the 1937

Census of Unemployment. To encourage people to participate in this census, Roosevelt spoke to Americans through the radio in one of his fireside chats.[28]

Finally, as part of Roosevelt's Works Progress Administration (WPA), a systematic procedure was set up to collect unemployment data in 1940 and was called the Current Population Survey (CPS). Those at the WPA argued that taking a census—that is, asking everyone about their employment status—was too time-consuming and too expensive to do frequently.[106] Therefore, only a subset of residents (a sample) would be surveyed in the CPS instead of everyone in the country (a census).

The federal government still uses this survey today, and it's the same one which is used to calculate the labor force participation rate. In the CPS, 60,000 households are in the sample at any given time. Households are selected to represent the entirety of the U.S., both rural and urban. For reliability reasons, each household is surveyed by the Census Bureau multiple times across a few months.

The people surveyed within each household are asked about their employment status, among other things. If they aren't currently working, they are asked what types of things (if any) they have done to find a job within the previous four weeks.[32]

In addition to collecting data from households, BLS contacts nearly 150,000 business and governmental agencies (who employ people too!) every month. As these organizations may have offices in multiple locations, the survey ends up including almost 700,000 worksites around the country.[25] This survey is called the Current Employment Statistics (CES) program.

The CES gathers information on wages and salaries, hours worked, and so forth, which supplements the unemployment and labor force information provided by CPS.[16] All of this information is rolled into "The Employment Situation."

Pheww. Now that we've reached modern times, let's look at how these surveys help to produce unemployment statistics.

POSSIBILITIES FOR U

Every month, people wait eagerly for the economic news contained in "The Employment Situation," or, more colloquially, the monthly jobs report. While the report is lengthy, two numbers immediately ricochet around the media, the stock markets, and in politicians' speeches: (a) the number of jobs added and (b) the unemployment rate. These numbers often turn into a mini-referendum on an administration's policies.

To calculate these statistics, CPS sorts people who are 16 years or older who are neither in the military nor institutionalized (e.g., prison, nursing home) into six categories (this is "everyone" from our labor force participation rate definitions):

1. people working full-time,

2. people happy working part-time,

3. people working part-time but who would rather work full-time,

4. people not working, but have been looking for a job in the past four weeks,

5. people not working and would like to, but are not actively looking for a job (this includes people who quit looking for a job because they became discouraged), and

6. everyone else who is not looking for a job.

The unemployment rate is the number of people considered unemployed divided by the number of people in the labor force. There is not just one unemployment measure but six, charmingly named U1 to U6. Who counts as unemployed and who counts as the labor force depends on the categories above.[32]

U1 measures long-term unemployment. U2 tracks people who either just lost their job or finished a temporary one. That is, U2 zooms in on the newly-unemployed.

The official unemployment rate is U3. The labor force consists of the first four categories in the list, the fourth group representing the unemployed. (The labor force participation rate is calculated from this definition of the labor force.)

Moving from U3 to U6, we steadily absorb more people into the labor force and classify more people as unemployed. This is visible when comparing U3 and U6 in Figure 2.2. The boxes correspond to the six divisions of the population. The thick, black outline identifies those that comprise the labor force. Finally, the shaded boxes are those considered unemployed.

The most expansive definition of unemployment is U6, which includes everyone who would like a job but isn't currently looking for one—at least not in the last four weeks—to the labor force.

U3 Statistic

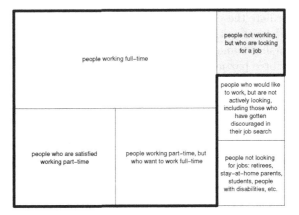

U6 Statistic

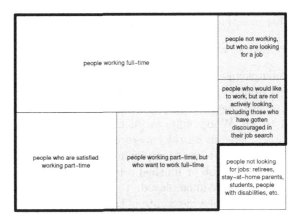

Figure 2.2 The full rectangle represents everyone who is 16 or older, not in the military, and not institutionalized. These people are then divided into six categories which are the boxes within the rectangle. The U3 and U6 statistics drawn here are the most commonly reported unemployment rates, computed as the ratio of unemployed people to the size of the labor force. Here, the thick, black outline represents the labor force and the shaded box(es) represent the unemployed. (Source: Bureau of Labor Statistics.)

U.S. Unemployment Rate

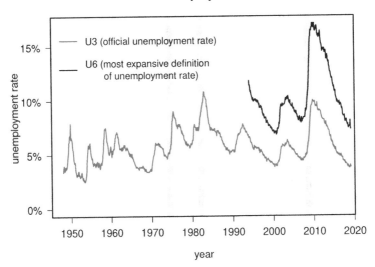

Figure 2.3 Monthly, seasonally adjusted U.S. unemployment rates using the U3 (blue) and U6 (black) definitions. The shaded areas represent the major recessions in the U.S.: after the 1973 and 1979 oil crises and the Great Recession. (Sources: Current Population Survey; National Bureau of Economic Research.)

Moreover, who counts as unemployed is larger as well: those who want a job regardless of whether they are looking for one along with those who are working part-time but want a full-time job.

While U3 can be calculated back to 1948, U6 appeared only in 1994. (Various U-monikered statistics existed before 1994, but their definitions differed from those in use today.)

We can compare seasonally adjusted U3 and U6 statistics in Figure 2.3. (This is another example of a time series graph.) Remember that seasonal adjustment means we've smoothed out the bumps so that we can better see general trends over time.

The first feature which jumps out is that U6 is always higher than U3; the second is that they move in tandem. We also see that unemployment is never zero. We need some unemployment to account for people switching jobs or entering the job market. Therefore, what economists consider "full employment" generally involves a non-zero unemployment rate.

We can also see that both U3 and U6 soared during each recession. What is interesting is that the gap between U3 and U6 widened substantially during the last recession. And so, we will focus next on people counted as unemployed in U6, but not in U3.

WHAT'S IN A NAME?

Not all jobs are created equal. Some jobs require a lot of training, others do not. Some jobs have regular hours whereas others are assigned at the last minute. One effect of counting jobs is they are treated equally. Employed? Great. Unemployed? Not great. However, that obscures the variety of jobs which exist in an economy. Tomato pickers. Lawyers. Waiters. Teachers. Photographers.

Jobs have different remuneration schemes as well. From regular salaries to hourly wages. From zero-hour contracts to internships. Treating them the same way when computing labor statistics papers over these differences. Whether or not people are making a living wage is irrelevant.

A primary division between types of jobs is between full-time and part-time work. For the latter, a key question is why people are only working part-time. In CPS, these people are split into various categories, three of which we will focus on here. First, some people decide to work fewer hours "by choice." That could mean they are taking care of children or sick relatives, are in school, or simply want to work part-time. The second and third groups are comprised of those with part-time jobs, but would rather be working full-time. Some part-timers couldn't find a full-time one whereas others have reduced hours because of "unfavorable business conditions."

In Figure 2.4, we can compare these three groups from 1955 to 2019.[19] We are focusing only on people who do not work on a farm (i.e., non-agricultural) because such work is heavily seasonal, subject to other rules, and is therefore often in its own category.

Nearly 80% of part-time workers say they work fewer hours by choice. However, the most interesting aspect of this graph is what happened after the housing bubble burst in 2007. There was a sharp increase in the percentage of part-timers who had their hours cut (black line). It is possible (though we are speculating here) that these individuals were previously working full-time and

Types of Non–Agricultural Part–Time Workers

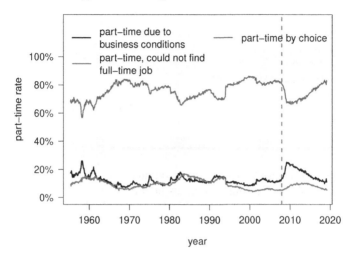

Figure 2.4   Three types of part-time, non-agricultural workers are graphed here: those who were part-time by choice (gray); those who work part-time because of forced reduced hours and other kinds of business conditions (black); and those who were unable to find full-time work (blue). The percentage in each category is graphed with the start of the great recession marked. This monthly data has been seasonally adjusted. (Sources: Current Population Survey; National Bureau of Economic Research.)

suddenly found themselves working part-time instead. As the economy improved, this percentage slowly decreased.

This is one benefit of having multiple unemployment measures. U3 would count everyone in Figure 2.4 as employed, even though some of them may not be happy with their circumstances. U6, however, distinguishes between these types of part-time workers.

With the rise of the gig economy, the nature of employment is shifting. People who work at these types of jobs, such as a driver for Uber or someone on a temporary contract, are technically called "contingent workers." We may need new types of U statistics in the future to learn more about these types of workers.

WE EXPECT 110% PERCENT

Shoveling,
Wrecking,
Planning,
Building, breaking, rebuilding

Carl Sandburg, 1914
Chicago

Industriousness is a celebrated quality in a capitalist society, as this line from Sandburg's famous poem reflects.[135] Accordingly, there are many ardent debates about why people don't have a job. For starters, the Industrial Revolution began replacing many jobs done by humans with machines. On the optimistic side, economist John Maynard Keynes wrote in 1930 that "technological unemployment" was temporary.[89] Eventually, he reasoned, it would be replaced by people working fewer hours and spending their free time on artistic pursuits. The chase for larger piles of money would end!

The other end of this discussion veered into murky areas of who *ought* to be working and why they were not doing so. A WPA employee observed that people often disparagingly claimed that, "Anyone who really wants a job can find one." Others enquired why a person experienced what was uncharitably called a "period of idleness."[156]

The reasons for people being out of work are often more complicated than being lazy. Some possible explanations from the 1930 census include:[27]

voluntary lay-off	plant closed
personal disability	part-time
family reasons	substitute workers
weather conditions	machines introduced
breakdown	reduction of force
off-season	cheaper labor substituted
lack of orders	worker too old
job completed	laid off
shortage of materials	dissatisfaction

The length of this list is a good sign as it incorporates a wide range of plausible reasons for being unemployed. There is, however, a critical problem: The jobless person is self-diagnosing his reason for being unemployed. Therefore, many of these choices are purely speculative, leaving ample room for inaccurate results. And so, by 1945, those probing questions were dropped from the surveys.[28] Now, people are only asked if they would like a job. If so, they are asked if they are "available to work" and whether they have given up looking for a job. The advantage these questions have is they are clear. The downside (and this is a big downside) is they provide little information about an important group.

The U3 statistic omits two groups of people from the labor force: those who aren't looking for a job (e.g., retired, studying, disabled) and those who want a job but aren't actively looking. We focus on the latter bunch in Figure 2.5.

Figure 2.5A shows that in 1995, around 10% of the people U3 drops from the labor force are those who want a job but aren't actually searching for one. While that percentage has generally been falling, we can see an uptick during the Great Recession after the burst of the 2007 housing bubble.

We can look at a subset of this group more closely in Figure 2.5B. Here, those who gave up on their job search are graphed as a percentage of those who want a job. Before 2007, this statistic fluctuated around 7%, but after that point it shot up to 22%. Thanks to the subsequent recession, some of these people probably lost their job and then, disheartened, quit looking for a new one.

From a measurement perspective, these are people who stopped being counted in U3 once they gave up looking for a job. Handily, these individuals are then picked up in U6.

AROUND THE WORLD

The International Labour Organization (ILO) was launched as part of the Treaty of Versailles after World War I in 1919. It was eventually absorbed into the United Nations after World War II.

The ILO has many missions. For example, it works to ensure people have living wages and to improve working conditions. It also publishes manuals to help countries produce their own official statistics.

The ILO proposes a statistic similar to U3, counting as unemployed only people at least 15 years old who are not working but looking for a job. Many countries have adopted a similar measure.

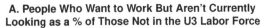

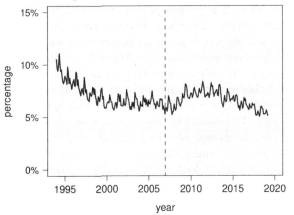

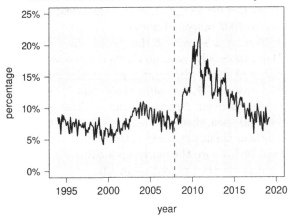

Figure 2.5 Plot A shows the percentage of people who want a job among those not counted as part of the U3 labor force. Plot B shows the percentage of people who have given up looking for a job among those from the group in Plot A. The data is not seasonally adjusted and was collected monthly. The start of the Great Recession is marked with the dotted line. (Sources: Current Population Survey; National Bureau of Economic Research.)

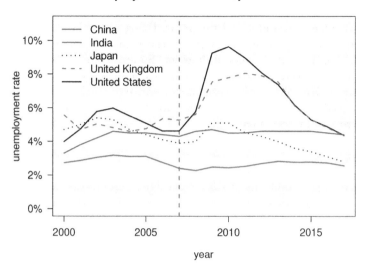

Unemployment Rate for People 15 and Over

Figure 2.6 Annual unemployment rate for five countries calculated using statistical models. The start of the Great Recession in the U.S. is marked. (Sources: © 2019 International Labour Organization, ILOSTAT; National Bureau of Economic Research.)

The United Kingdom and Japan, for example, both use the 15 years and older threshold for their unemployment rates; the U.S., as we've seen, starts its count at 16 years. (The minimum age is 16 in the U.S. because of child labor laws and schooling requirements.[16])

These differences in definitions can make it hard to compare unemployment rates across countries. Consequently, the ILO attempts to create comparable statistics by adjusting annual unemployment rates reported from different countries using additional demographic information with statistical models.

We can see its estimates in Figure 2.6 for five countries: the U.S. (our comparison point), China, India, Japan, and the United Kingdom. The U.S. unemployment rate is the most rocky. In particular, the unemployment rate roughly doubles after the 2007 crisis in the

U.S. and the United Kingdom compared to the Asian countries in our graph.[86]

These are very different nations, with very different governmental structures and social programs. Being unemployed in the U.S. differs from not having a job in the United Kingdom or in India. Working conditions are different. So are labor protections. Moreover, for those who are counted as employed, we can't tell whether those jobs pay a living wage, are temporary, or require specialized skills. We need to make sure we don't read too much into cross-country comparisons.

SUMMARY

Widespread unemployment during the Great Depression spurred the federal government to track the unemployment rate on a regular basis. As a result, every month since 1948, the official unemployment statistic—or U3—is reported as part of the closely monitored "The Employment Situation."

U3, one of six unemployment measures, is the ratio of the unemployed to the labor force and is considered a lagging economic indicator. Only people who do not have a job and have been looking for one in the past four weeks are counted as unemployed. The labor force participation rate is the ratio of people in the labor force to the total number of potential workers.

The various statistics in "The Employment Situation" are published by the Bureau of Labor Statistics using the Current Population Survey and the Current Employment Statistics program. These include the labor force participation rate and the number of jobs created, in addition to the unemployment rate.

FURTHER READING

Glass House: The 1% Economy and the Shattering of the All-American Town by Brian Alexander. St. Martin's Press, 2017.

The Hocking Glass Company opened in 1905 in Lancaster, a small town in Ohio. Its executives lived in town and their wives volunteered in the local community. Moreover, its workers had dependable manufacturing jobs and their children went to good schools. In 1947, Forbes regaled it as the "all-American town." As this book's title implies, this idyll no longer exists. Alexander, who grew up in Lancaster, recounts with painstaking and distressing detail the town's decline. This decay occurred after multiple leveraged buyouts spliced the company's managers from its workers. The critical insight here is that the popular narrative of manufacturing being shifted overseas was not the cause of this town's collapse.

Factory Girls: From Village to City in a Changing China by Leslie T. Chang. Spiegel & Grau, 2008.

More than 130 million people have moved to factory cities from rural communities in the past few decades, marking a major shift in Chinese society. This ethnography describes the harsh lives and warm hopes of the women who work in factories making everything from athletic shoes to mobile phones. Through the stories of individual women, Chang offers a humanizing look at the issues of outsourcing and the global employment market. Within this narrative, the author weaves her own family history of migration and loss.

Fireside Chat on the Unemployment Census by Franklin D. Roosevelt, 1937.

This transcript forms part of President Franklin D. Roosevelt's radio series of "Fireside Chats" with the American public. In this one, given in November of 1937, he encourages people to fill out the Census of Unemployment (this was different from the decennial census). He explains in a folksy manner how he wants to use the "fact-seeking census" to find ways to get people back to work. He ends by emphasizing that idle or underpaid workers mean fewer consumers.

CHAPTER 3

Inequality

THE BOOK OF GENESIS, Chapter 13 of the Bible recounts a story involving Abraham and Lot. Having fled Egypt, the two men find that their new settlement is unable to support both families' cattle. Abraham suggests a solution, "Is not the whole land before you? Separate yourself from me. If you take the left hand, then I will go to the right; or if you take the right hand, then I will go to the left" (Gen. 13:9 (NSRV)[109]). Lot agrees and heads to the plain of Jordan, leaving Abraham to reside in Canaan.

The modern—albeit less solemn—counterpart to Abraham's proposal is the cake-sharing problem. Let's say you and a friend plan to share a cake, a pie, or a pizza. You partition it, and your friend chooses which slice she wants. You take what's left.

Solving an inequality problem this way appeals to an innate sense of fairness and attempts to mitigate any subsequent jealousy. The goal is to attain an equitable division.

Moving away from desserts to slicing the proverbial "economic pie," our notion of equity may shift. Whether this fairness principle still applies is up for debate. At the extremes, it may still be appropriate. It hardly seems fair for one person to have all of the money. On the other hand, imagine income is distributed evenly among everyone. Many people—especially those who feel like they're working harder—would undoubtedly object.

When the global financial crisis hit in the late 2000s, everyone started talking about inequality, particularly income inequality. People made comparisons to the Gilded Age. Occupy Wall Street protestors demonstrated. Authors wrote a slew of articles and books attempting to explain "how we got here" and "how to fix it." Politicians absorbed the buzzword into their stump speeches.

These inequities at the societal level invariably invoke discussions on weighty topics such as equality, liberty, social mobility, and personal responsibility. Even defining these terms is fraught—for example, when talking about "equality" one person may be talking about equality of outcomes, another about opportunity, and a third about both.

When economists tackle these questions, they like to have something to measure. This gives them a way to describe a phenomenon. And one place to start is to ask a big, bald question: Who makes the most?

CEO VS. EMPLOYEES

One rough gauge of inequality is to compare the annual salary of CEOs—the bosses—to the money earned by "average workers." There is an intuitive appeal to this approach: We picture CEOs as rich and workers as not so rich.

We read the "CEO versus average worker" statistics often in the press. The headlines cut straight to the point: "Top CEOs make more than 300 times the average worker," ran a headline in *Fortune* in June 2015.[82] "Report: CEOs Earn 331 Times As Much As Average Workers, 774 Times As Much As Minimum Wage Earners," *Forbes* reported in April 2014.[63]

But wait: In May 2015, again in *Forbes*, a different columnist reported, "The Average CEO Makes Four Times The Average Worker."[162]

The big point is consistent and obvious: CEOs make more money. But how much more? Is it 774 times, 331 times, four times, or some other number? The answer is, it depends on whom you ask, and how you ask.

The conflicting headlines pull numbers from two studies, each published by different organizations that were, nonetheless, looking at the same data:

- The American Federation of Labor and Congress of Industrial Organizations (AFL–CIO)—which comprises national and international unions—estimated the ratio at 373 to 1.[4]

- The other study, published by the American Enterprise Institute (AEI), a nonprofit think tank, reported the ratio at 4.6 to 1.[123]

That's a pretty big disparity. To explain it, we need definitions for the terms worker, CEO, and compensation.

Let's start with average workers. Both the AFL–CIO and AEI base their claims on data published by the Bureau of Labor Statistics (BLS). BLS aggregates employment data collected through the Current Employment Statistics survey. Every month, the survey releases data on things like employment, hours worked, and earnings based on a sample from a list of 9.7 million businesses, which is thought to cover 97 percent of all employed people in the U.S.[24] (This survey should sound familiar; we talked about it in the jobs chapter.)

The survey covers more than 800 different jobs from computer programmers to tour guides to bookbinders. However, for our analysis, there are only two categories: CEOs and everyone else.

The AFL–CIO report treats "everyone else" as people who are not managers or bosses. When they did their analysis in 2014, these people earned an average of $36,314 annually. The AEI takes a different approach. They include bosses and managers in their "everyone else" category, arriving at an average annual salary of $47,230. The AEI value is considerably higher because—as you've already guessed—it includes managers and other executive types who make around $112,500 per year.

We've already picked up some of the disparity, but not enough to account for the radical difference in income ratios.

To figure out CEO compensation, we have to break down both terms—"CEO" and "compensation." The AEI study reported that the more than 20,000 CEOs in the U.S. made, on average, $216,100 per year in 2014. That's gross pay, which is their official salary and generally does not include bonuses or other perks. The AFL–CIO report includes only 472 CEOs from businesses listed in the Standard & Poor's 500 Index (S&P 500®). This is an index of the largest public companies in the U.S. like Walmart, American Airlines, Facebook, Aetna, and J.P. Morgan Chase.

Big companies submit employment data to the Securities and Exchange Commission (SEC), a government watchdog of the stock market. When these firms submit their CEO compensation numbers, they include things like stock options and bonuses. The AFL–CIO used these SEC documents to determine that the average CEO compensation was $13.5 million annually.

This discrepancy between the AFL–CIO and AEI values accounts for most of the difference between the final numbers.

The third question is the same for both studies. In both cases, the ratio is computed by taking the average pay for CEOs across firms divided by the average worker pay across firms. The calculations are easy; it's the definitions that cause trouble. The AFL–CIO value makes it look like the U.S. is extremely unequal, whereas the AEI value indicates the opposite. The sheer magnitude of 373 to 1 made the first number popular in the media.[4]

In the end, however, neither method would work for an official estimate of inequality. Ignore the headlines. If we take a step back, we might want to ask why we focus so intently on CEOs in the first place.

Maybe CEOs are appealing because they're a proxy for the mega-rich: Warren Buffett, Steve Jobs, Bill Gates. We even read about their compensation in the news: Jamie Dimon at J.P. Morgan Chase was paid $18.2 million in 2015, Lloyd Blankfein at Goldman Sachs made $22.6 million, and Indra Nooyi at PepsiCo earned $26.4 million.[95]

Newspaper articles dive into the reasons for such lucrative pay, from the public venerating the solo exploits of top CEOs to a corporate edition of "keeping up with the Joneses."[91, 101] But in terms of understanding our inequality measures, the CEO is really a stand-in for the general population of high earners like athletes and movie stars. It's an idea that's accessible to everyone—even though, logically, analyzing the compensation of 500 people out of 324 million in the U.S. may not give us a complete snapshot.

Here's another issue: Not all companies are the same. The labor survey lists 840 occupations, but they don't exist in every company. Financial firms don't keep construction workers on the payroll; graphic design companies don't need phlebotomists. How money is spent can vary dramatically among companies by virtue of being in different fields; some need reserves for research and development, others for purchasing raw materials or shipping cargo.

A better way to compute the statistic we want—that is, something to quantify inequality—is to calculate it not across all firms, everywhere, but within an individual firm itself.

In the AFL–CIO and AEI measures, the average income was calculated by taking the average of all the workers, no matter where they worked or what they did. (This decision was a practical one based on the types of information available to both organizations.)

We'll get a more interesting measure if, instead, we start by calculating the average salary within a company. Then, we can calculate the ratio of CEO pay to average worker pay—also within the company. Keeping in mind variables like company size, we can compare ratios across companies.

In this revised version, a single ratio gives us information about inequality in one firm; comparing ratios across firms gives us (limited) information on inequality in the economy.

Understanding inequality is a timely pursuit: In 2007, what later became known as the Great Recession began to ripple through the U.S. The housing market bubble burst was followed by a financial crisis and the issue of income inequality became a prominent topic. Many people worried that good jobs in manufacturing and coal mining were being shipped overseas, replaced by robots, or being lost to emerging industries elsewhere. Donald J. Trump made this a hot topic on the campaign trail and ultimately won the 2016 U.S. presidential election.

Also in 2016, Stanford University published the results of a study which examined how the American population viewed CEOs at major corporations. They found 66% of Democrats, 52% of Republicans, and 64% of Independents felt, "there is a maximum amount that a CEO should be paid relative to the average worker, no matter the company and its performance." Furthermore, they estimated that nearly half of the population felt that the government should enact policies to curb CEO pay.[93]

There have been efforts to do just that. In 2010, during President Barack Obama's administration, Congress passed the Dodd–Frank Wall Street Reform and Consumer Protection Act (i.e., Dodd-Frank), which tried to impose regulations designed to prevent another financial crisis. It required large, publicly-traded companies to disclose the ratio of CEO pay to median worker pay.[137] That provision was designed to give shareholders information about the company; another goal, in effect, was to help reduce income inequality one firm at a time.

Sound familiar?

The CEO pay ratio required by Dodd–Frank is a within-company version of the AEI statistic. The only difference is that median pay is used instead of average pay.

The median is the number that you find in the middle of a list of numbers, if you line them up from lowest to highest. To see how it affects the statistic, imagine a company—we'll call it Firm A—that has a CEO and five other employees. The annual salaries of the non-CEO employees are listed below from lowest to highest.

Firm A: $25,000 $30,000 $50,000 $70,000 $120,000

The number in the middle is $50,000 and that's the median salary. The average, which we get by adding all the salaries and dividing by 5, is $59,000. These two numbers are close. Now, let's look at Firm B, which also has five employees working under the CEO:

Firm B: $25,000 $30,000 $50,000 $70,000 $1,000,000

Here, the median salary is still $50,000, but the average has ballooned to $235,000!

The median is again determined by the middle value, so a few very large or very small salaries will not affect the result, provided that the ordering of the salaries does not change substantially. The average, on the other hand, is extremely sensitive to the magnitude of these salaries. The one person who makes $1,000,000 in Firm B pulls the average salary up, making it seem as if the typical salary for all employees is very high, even though no one else makes anywhere close to the average.

The million dollar employee would be considered an outlier; that is, an extreme person compared to the other employees in the company. Outliers have a larger impact on the average than the median, which, in technical terms, says that the average is a less robust measure of center than the median.

Incomes in the real world generally look more like Firm B than Firm A. That is, a few people make a lot more money than everyone else. This is the crux of income inequality, of course, but as a result the median is a more accurate reflection of the "typical" worker salary than the average. And so, because of outliers, the use of median pay in the CEO pay ratio is better than using the average pay. (Again, provided you have access to median pay.)

The Dodd–Frank rule, barring the murkiness associated with who counts as an employee (e.g., foreign versus domestic, full-time versus contractor), is the best version of the CEO pay ratio statistic, broad-brush though it may be.

THE 1%

On December 15th, 1989, a 7,100 pound bronze bull appeared in front of the New York Stock Exchange. It was a mischievous Christmas surprise sculpted by artist Arturo Di Modica and was a representation of the might of the American.[100] The police, unamused and unimpressed, hauled the heavy bovine to an impound lot because Di Modica had neglected to secure a permit. Popular demand prevailed, though, and the bull came back less than a week later, reinstalled in the north end of nearby Bowling Green Park.[6] The Charging Bull has since remained a popular destination among tourists, some of whom, inexplicably, rub the bull's soccer ball-sized testicles for good luck.

Here was a sculpture which represented the recovery of the U.S. economy after the stock market crash of 1987, a positive symbol of the American success story. But two decades later, the financial crisis hit the economy, resulting in a sharp reversal in this bull's significance.

On September 17th, 2011, demonstrators planned to gather around the Charging Bull to protest against rising inequality. The bull now represented hubris rather than strength. Police barricaded the sculpture and the protesters made their way toward Zucotti Park, sparking what became a global movement: Occupy Wall Street.[122] Their slogan, "We Are the 99 Percent," spoke to the idea that 1% of people control an unfair share of income and, perhaps more importantly, wealth. (Income is how much money you earn; wealth is the value of the stuff you own—car, house, furniture, stocks, etc.) This idea has become a potent symbol for the growing inequality within the country. Bernie Sanders even channeled the movement into a bid for President of the United States in 2016.

Occupy Wall Street gives us another opportunity to look at an inequality metric—and another chance to work through a back-of-the-envelope calculation. This time, we want to know what percentage of wealth is actually held by the top 1%.

On the global scale, the top 1% of adults on the planet controlled roughly 47% of wealth in mid-2018. With total wealth estimated to be nearly $317 trillion at the current exchange rate—that is, $317,000,000,000,000—47% is a large amount whose scale is hard to truly comprehend.[140] A lot of money is (still) held by not very many people.

Pitting the 1% against the 99% is nearly as dramatic as pitting the CEO against "Average Joe." This characteristic makes the statistic an appealing soundbite. However, 1% is an extremely small sliver of the world's adults. In 2018, a person would need to have net assets of $871,320 to join this exclusive club.[140] (You can calculate your net assets by taking the value of everything you own, and subtracting your debt and other liabilities.)

Maybe we should look at the top 10% instead, a group with decidedly less headline appeal, but more people. People can be admitted into that group with \$93,170 in assets—a big drop from the 1 percenters.[140] It is easy to imagine that some people in the 1% are staggeringly wealthy. (You don't even have to imagine; you can just click through *Forbes'* annual list of billionaires.) The 10%, on the other hand, includes people who would not be considered wealthy in many countries.

This leads us to an even more sobering statistic: the top 10% of the global population holds 85% of the wealth.[140] By adding just a few more people to the top group, we have covered nearly all of the wealth on the planet! Like the 1%, the wealth controlled by the 10% has also been climbing.[126]

One advantage of talking about inequality this way is that it avoids what was an arbitrary dividing line between CEOs and those lumped together as everyone else. This is because not all top earners are CEOs and not all CEOs are top earners. The CEO statistic fails to give us a clear idea regarding inequality since it is not an expedient way of separating high earners from everyone else. Ranking people by earnings as opposed to grouping by occupation produces a less ambiguous statistic. A short example will explain why.

Imagine a hypothetical population of 100 people, including 14 people who are CEOs. Our goal is to compare the pay of CEOs with the pay of people in the top 10%.

Figure 3.1 presents the income for each person in our imaginary society. We place the individual with the lowest income on the left and continue in rank order to the person with the highest income on the right. Each bar on this graph represents one person in the population and the height of each bar is their income.

From this graph, we see that incomes range from around \$5,000 per year to more than \$1 million per year. To make the following discussion easier, a dotted horizontal line at \$225,000 and a vertical dotted line to identify the cutoff for the top 10% have been added to the graph.

To calculate the fraction of income earned by the top 10%, we only have to add up the heights of those 10 bars and divide by the total income for the whole population. (If we wanted to study the top 1%, we'd take a similar approach, dividing the height of the highest bar by the total income.)

You'll notice that some of those bars are colored blue—those are our 14 CEOs. Some of them made the top 10; some didn't. It is now immediately apparent that the very top earners are not all CEOs. The reverse is true as well.

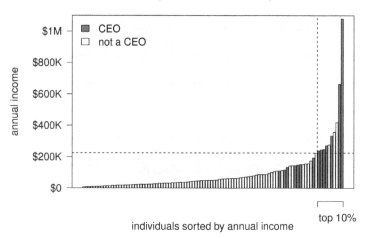

Figure 3.1 Comparing CEOs with those in the top 10% who earn $225,000 or more in an imaginary society.

There's a tradeoff here between CEO pay and the top percent statistics. What the 10% statistic (and the 1% version) gives up in terms of approachability (it's easy to visualize a caricature CEO) it gains in usability.

In contrast to CEO pay ratio, we mostly have been focusing here on measuring wealth instead of income. Wealth, is essentially, a person's assets (money in the bank, home equity) with their liabilities (credit card debt, remaining mortgage payments) subtracted. Income refers only to money being accrued, like a person's salary, interest from a bank account, or profit from a home sale.

Figure 3.2 shows how the estimated shares of income and wealth of the top 10 % in the United States have changed since 1960. (Note that the share of wealth is always higher than the share of income. This is unsurprising as wealth can be accumulated over many years and later inherited by the next generation.)

Step by step, we're gaining a more precise measure of inequality. We started this section with the 1%, then expanded our analysis to include the top 10%. This gives us an idea of what's happening with some of the people in a population, but not everyone. We don't know how income (or wealth) is distributed among the other

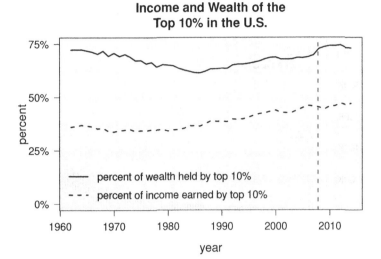

Figure 3.2 Comparing wealth (solid line) and income (dotted line) estimates for the top 10% in the United States across the past few decades. The vertical line marks the beginning of the Great Recession in December 2007. (Sources: World Inequality Database; National Bureau of Economic Research.)

90% or 40% or 60%. One step toward a granular understanding is to study income and wealth by *deciles*.

There's a good chance you've encountered deciles before. If you plan to attend, do attend, or attended college in the U.S., you probably took the SAT—a multiple choice rite-of-passage that focuses on reading comprehension, math, and possibly writing. Your results would have included a score and a percentile. The latter tells you how your score compares to everyone else who took the test. If you scored at the 90th percentile, for example, then your score was at least as high as 90% of the other test-takers. Another way to say that is you're in the 10th decile, or top 10%. The higher the percentile, the better you scored compared to all of the other test-takers.

(If we convert the percent to a decimal, this would be called a quantile in statistics. For example, the 50th percentile would be the 0.5 quantile and says that 50% of test-takers earned the same SAT score as you or lower. This is the formal definition of the median which was discussed in the CEO pay ratio section of this chapter.) Now apply that same idea to income and wealth. First, sort everyone by income, lowest to highest. The 10% of the population with the lowest incomes make up the first decile. The 10% of population with the highest incomes would make up the tenth decile. (Everyone to the right of the dotted vertical line in Figure 3.1 would be in the tenth decile.)

To land in the tenth decile in 2014, you had to have earned more than $118,215 that year. That means 90% of earners in the U.S. made $118,215 or less. We can learn more by looking at the percentage of income earned by each decile. In 2014, for example, the top 10%—tenth decile—of earners took home 47.02% of all income and held 72.98% of all wealth in the U.S.[161]

Conversely, we can ask what percentage of income was earned by the first decile (lowest 10% of earners), or fifth decile, or whichever decile we want. This way, we can learn more about other segments of society. In Table 3.3, you can see wealth and income in the U.S. in 2014, broken down by decile.

Perhaps the most glaring numbers in the table are the first two in the wealth column because they are both negative. This tells us that the bottom 20%—the first and second decile—had debts exceeding their total assets. The people in this group are not necessarily the same individuals who are in the bottom 20% of income earners, so we can't say anything more about them. That is, we don't know why their debts outweigh their assets: maybe they just bought a house, or have high balances on credit cards.

Data like these let us track economic changes; for example, we might look at how people in the lower deciles fared during and after the Great Recession (December 2007 through June 2009).[108] Look back at Figure 3.2 for a second—you'll see that the recession (marked by a vertical dotted line) barely perturbed the income share of the top 10%, and didn't stop the upward climb of their share of wealth. The top graph in Figure 3.4 shows how things changed for people—markedly for the worse—in the lower deciles within the same time period.

People in the lowest decile have a negative share for the entire duration, showing that they have more debt than assets. But in the wake of the financial crisis, that debt increases sharply—shown by the plummeting graph representing wealth.

A similar pattern of increasing debt holds with those in the 2nd decile, but to a lesser degree. Things become even more downcast

TABLE 3.3   Wealth and income percentage estimates by
decile for the U.S. in 2014. Negative values for wealth
indicate that debts exceeded assets for at least some
individuals within that decile. Note that the cumulative
income column does not equal 100% due to rounding.
(Source: World Inequality Database.)

Decile	% Wealth	Cum. % Wealth	% Income	Cum. % Income
1	-1.23	-1.23	0.19	0.19
2	-0.34	-1.57	1.49	1.68
3	0.01	-1.56	2.48	4.16
4	0.28	-1.28	3.55	7.71
5	1.15	-0.13	4.82	12.53
6	2.25	2.12	6.40	18.93
7	4.10	6.22	8.29	27.22
8	7.35	13.57	10.77	37.99
9	13.45	27.02	14.98	52.97
10	72.98	100.00	47.02	99.99

when we look at what happens to people in the 3rd decile: Their
share of wealth tracked positive until 2008, when it dropped below
zero and into the red.

These three deciles comprise 30% of the adult population,
around 70 million individuals! The recession, clearly, was painful
for these people.

If we look at income earned rather than wealth held, we can
see more stark differences divided along deciles. Look at the dotted
line in Figure 3.2: The percentage of income earned by the top 10%
has slowly increased across decades. The opposite is true for the
lower deciles, which we can see in the second plot in Figure 3.4.

In all three cases, after a brief upward bump in the early 1960s,
the general trend in the share of income has been downwards.
(Since income includes both wages and salaries along with capital gains, there are many moving parts. This graph does not tell
us which components of income have changed over time within a
decile and so we cannot explain this trend from the graph alone.)

Joseph Stiglitz, who won the 2001 Nobel Prize in Economics,
grew up in Gary, Indiana. This was once a booming steel town on
the shores of Lake Michigan. In interviews, he recalls seeing the
town rife with discrimination, inequality, and unemployment—a
system that benefitted only a select few. These experiences moti-
vated his research on the causes and effects of inequality.

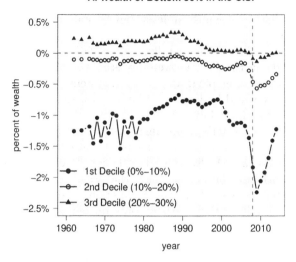

A. Wealth of Bottom 30% in the U.S.

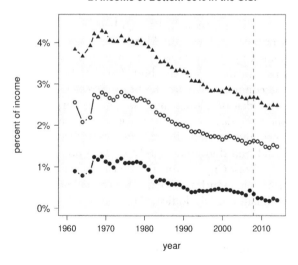

B. Income of Bottom 30% in the U.S.

Figure 3.4 Wealth and income for the lower three deciles are shown. The vertical lines mark the start of the Great Recession; the horizontal line at 0 in plot A indicates the point above which assets exceed debt. (Sources: World Inequality Database; National Bureau of Economic Research.)

He showed that recent financial increases among those at the top have come mostly from capital gains rather than salary increases, the latter of which at least can be indicative of worker productivity.

We started off this chapter talking about fair ways of division, but we could—in theory—sidestep discussions about the fairness of slicing the economic pie if we imagine a system where the pie is continuously replaced by larger and larger pies. At the very least, everyone's lot is improving.

But that's not what's happening. Instead, we see those with the largest slices increasing their share at the expense of those individuals who have the least. Stiglitz thought that governmental policies incentivized the 1% to behave that way.[147]

The patterns we see from the calculations and graphs we've studied so far tell us that focusing only on one segment of the population—whether the top 1% or a particular decile—is insufficient to fully understand inequality.

The story is far more complex. Even the CEO pay ratio statistic included information about the "average worker." To fix this problem, we turn to a third measure, the Gini coefficient.

Before we get there, though, let's go back to the bull on Wall Street for a curious epilogue. In March 2017, the Charging Bull statue was joined by the Fearless Girl—a bronze statue of a child, hands on hips, staring down the bull. Created by artist Kristen Visbal, it was commissioned by the State Street Global Advisors to promote the idea of adding more women to corporate boards. It was installed the day before International Women's Day, again giving new meaning to the bull.

The girl and bull duo immediately became popular (and infamous) and New York City Mayor, Bill de Blasio, extended Fearless Girl's stay from one month to a year. One can debate the merits of corporate feminism but Di Modica, the creator of the bull, was not a fan.[143] Neither was local artist Alex Gardega, who added a sculpture of an ugly dog urinating on Fearless Girl—enter the Pissing Pug. After three hours, Gardega removed the dog.[83] This bronze bull went from showing American strength to weakness, feminism to farce!

LORENZ AND GINI

In the previous section, we talked about comparing income and wealth by dividing a population into tenths, and comparing deciles.

It's a helpful way to think about the problem, but it can get burdensome quickly. And tough to keep track of.

It's hard to figure out what conclusions we can draw about inequality if the shares of wealth in the first and fourth deciles increase, but the third and sixth decrease. It's also hard to figure out how to compare these 10 numbers to the corresponding 10 in Japan or India.

Instead of assembling Table 3.3 on page 36 decile by decile, let us calculate cumulative amounts instead. We can use this to create an aggregate measure of inequality called the Gini coefficient. Two columns of the table illustrate how this would work by reporting the running total of the income percentage earned.

We start with 0.19, the percentage earned by the first decile. The second decile's income share is 1.49%, so we add that number to get a total of 1.68, and so on—until we reach the bottom of the table, which accounts for the full population. We should see 100% of income—which we do—because we are accounting for 100% of the population. (The percentages in the "% Income" column of Table 3.3 do not sum perfectly to 100% because the estimates were rounded when published.)

With this approach, we can see, for example, that 90% of the population earned 52.97% of the total income in 2014. And that the top 10% of the population earned the other 47%. Figure 3.5 shows a graphical version of the same cumulative data, each bar representing one row of the table. Each successive bar shows the cumulative income; the 9th bar—representing the bottom 9 deciles—has a height of 52.97%.

If we connect the height of those bars, we end up with an upward-sweeping curve. This is called a Lorenz curve. It's named after Max Otto Lorenz, who was born in Iowa in 1876 and later studied economics. Lorenz worked for various federal agencies including the Census Bureau and the Interstate Commerce Commission. He also directed the Eight-Hour Commission which studied the ramifications of the Adamson Act. This law instituted eight-hour workdays and other labor protections for railroad workers.[90]

In 1905 he published a paper introducing his curve with the twin goals of developing a method which could track inequality over time and allow for comparisons across countries.[97] (The first sentence of his paper is quoted at the beginning of this book.)

The "curve" in Figure 3.5 is choppy. If we divided up the population into smaller groups, such as batches of 5% or 1% instead

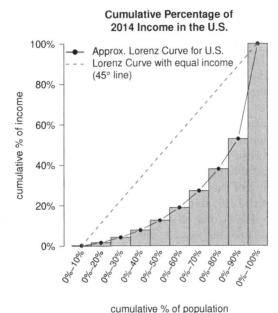

Figure 3.5 Bar graph of values in the fourth column of Table 3.3. Connecting the heights of each bar generates an approximate Lorenz curve (black). If everyone in the U.S. earned the same income, the Lorenz curve would be a 45° line (blue). (Source: World Inequality Database.)

of the 10% increments, Figure 3.5 would contain more bars and we would be connecting more dots to get our approximated curve.

If we increase the number of bars, our Lorenz curve would become more smooth—that is, more like an actual curve. Figure 3.6 shows the stylized version of such a curve.

We've been talking about income shares as percentages, but for our Lorenz curve graphs we'll convert those numbers into fractions—"shares"—so the vertical axis goes from 0 to 1, instead of 0 to 100.

If one person had all the income, then the Lorenz curve in Figure 3.6 would follow the horizontal axis until, at the very end, it would spike to 1. In contrast, if everyone had the same income, the bars would line up to yield a perfectly straight, 45° line.

Lorenz Curve

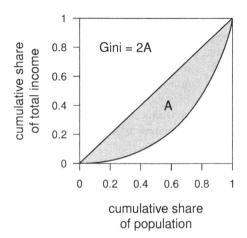

Figure 3.6 The Lorenz curve is the curved line in the graph above, from which the Gini coefficient is calculated. The region **A** corresponds to the area of the shaded section; twice that area equals the Gini coefficient.

Given how remote those possibilities are, Lorenz curves will usually look like some kind of swoop that falls beneath the 45° line. The area between the diagonal line and the Lorenz curve—marked **A** in Figure 3.6—represents the level of inequality. The larger the area **A**, the higher the inequality.

With the Lorenz curve, we can "see" inequality. By computing **A**, we can get a numerical estimate. Notice that the Lorenz curve sits in a box with sides of length 1, which means the area of the whole box is also 1. Half of that—the area under the diagonal—must be 1/2, which means the area of **A** will always be between 0 and 1/2.

It might be more helpful to recognize what *fraction* of the total area under the diagonal is occupied by **A**. This is actually a simple calculation. Since the total area is 1/2, the fraction is just **A** divided by 1/2, or 2 times the value of **A**.

This value—2 times A—is called the Gini coefficient. It captures inequality information about an entire population in one single number.

The Gini coefficient was named after Corrado Gini, who was an Italian contemporary of Lorenz and was born in 1884. Although he trained as a lawyer, his work as an academic and at the National Statistical Services in Italy was focused on statistics and its applications. He made significant contributions to the subject and had a singular dedication to his work.[77]

He had a dark side as president of two eugenics societies and some ambiguous connections to Mussolini.[90] Nevertheless, his eponymous statistic, which he termed the "concentration ratio," was published in 1914 sparking a new field which is still studied today.[77] Using the Lorenz curve is simply one way, out of many, to compute the Gini coefficient.

Here's what it looks like in practice. According to the Current Population Survey (CPS), the median annual income for households in 2017 was $51,372 and the Gini coefficient was 0.482. This gives us a little bit of information: 50% households earned below $51,372 and 50% of households earned above that amount.[37] (The survey also estimated a total of 127,586,000 households.)

There are many ways to divide total income so that we end up with a median of $51,372 across 127,586,000 households, but most of them do not yield the 2017 Gini coefficient of 0.482.

Figure 3.7 shows three examples with the same median income, but different Gini coefficients. In each of the hypothetical examples, we will assume the number of households and the median annual income matches the values published by CPS.

To start, let us say every household earned $51,372 annually. That means the average and median and highest and lowest incomes are identical. If we wanted to show this case graphically, like we did with our hypothetical population containing a few CEOs (see Figure 3.1), we would end up with 127,586,000 bars, each with the same height. This is tedious work for not much useful information.

Instead, we could use what is called a histogram. This type of graph was first introduced (and the word coined) by statistician Karl Pearson in 1891 during a series of lectures at Gresham College in England. His lessons were designed to be understood not only by fellow scientists, but also by laymen and so made full use of visual aids from charts and graphs to rolling dice and flipping coins.[99] (Unfortunately, like Gini, he too was involved in the eugenics movement.)

Histograms are a compact way to display quantitative data. In this simple case, our histogram is simply a single bar at $51,372

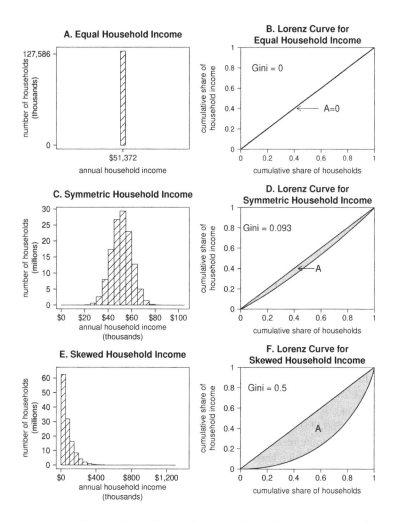

Figure 3.7 Three hypothetical examples of income distributions, each described with a histogram and corresponding Lorenz curve. Each income distribution has the same median annual income of $51,372 across 127,586,000 households. The Gini coefficient is twice the area of the region **A**, between the Lorenz curves and the diagonal line. (Source for 2017 median household income and number of households: 2018 Annual Social and Economic Supplement of the Current Population Survey.)

with a height of 127,586,000, the number of times this income occurs in the population. Figure 3.7A shows this.

Figure 3.7B shows the accompanying Lorenz curve. Since everyone earns the same amount, income accumulates evenly, and we end up with a diagonal line. The corresponding Gini coefficient is 0, because there's no area between the Lorenz curve and the diagonal line. That means no inequality. This system is unrealistic: No matter your years of experience and training, your income would be identical to everyone else's in this scenario.

Let's try again. The next row of the figure shows what would happen if income isn't always equal, but is distributed symmetrically. Visually, this just means that we can fold Figure 3.7C down the center and have (approximately) identical halves. For every household with a very low income, there is a high-earning one to balance it out. As in our first attempt, because of this symmetry, the mean and median annual household income would be approximately equal here at $51,372.

Also, like before, it is too time-consuming to plot every single income for the hundreds of millions of households, so now we'll group together incomes into ranges. (All households that made between $60,000 and $65,000 will be put into one group, those between $65,000 and $70,000 in another bucket, and so on.) The height of the bar corresponds to the number of households in that income range.

We can see that most households in this example seem to make between $50,000 and $70,000. Very few make less than $20,000 and even fewer make more than $100,000. That means the area of **A** is larger than 0. Twice the area of **A** generates our Gini coefficient of 0.089. Because it's so close to zero, we know inequality exists but is quite small in this example.

However, this is probably not a realistic case either. There are some people who have extremely high incomes (think Silicon Valley executives or Hollywood celebrities); the high-end of household income is limitless. This brings us to our final example, a skewed income distribution. In this case, we'll keep the median at $51,372, but we'll assume the high-earners earn a lot more money. Those high incomes, as we saw earlier, will pull the average higher, too.

Figure 3.7E shows our final histogram. It describes a population where most households have low annual incomes, since the highest bars are on the left. A few households have incomes that reach into the millions of dollars per year—they are on the right.

This dwindling string of stratospheric earners form what is called the tail of the distribution. In Figure 3.7E, you can see that there's no symmetry to this distribution; there's no matching of high earners to low earners. Instead, we call this shape skewed. (Since the tail heads out to the right, it is right-skewed.) You can imagine many examples of long tails: a few artists sell millions of albums, a few movies become blockbusters, a few books become bestsellers (hopefully this one!).

Using these incomes, we can construct the Lorenz curve in Figure 3.7F. Now, the area **A** is much larger than our earlier examples, indicating a much higher level of inequality in this population. In fact, the Gini coefficient is about 0.5 here—significantly higher than anything we've seen yet.

The examples in Figure 3.7 illustrate a few ways income could be distributed among a country's residents. In real life, however, income distributions tend to be right-skewed, the tail representing a few high earners.

PROS AND CONS

One advantage of the Gini coefficient is that it satisfies something called the Pigou–Dalton principle. It's easiest to illustrate this property with an example.

Let's say our friend Wilberforce earns $20,000 dollars per year, but Smitha earns $100,000 and Dongyu earns $80,000. All three live alone and therefore constitute their own households. Through some mechanism, $5,000 of Smitha's money goes to Wilberforce. Wilberforce may be richer, but he is still poorer than both Dongyu and Smitha. Moreover, Dongyu is still poorer than Smitha. Money may have shifted between Wilberforce and Smitha, but it hasn't changed the ranking of incomes.

The transfer of money makes the trio more equal and the Gini coefficient would decrease as a result. In general, if we can show that any transfer from a richer person to a poorer person which maintains the ranking of the incomes also decreases the inequality level, then the inequality measure upholds the Pigou–Dalton principle.

We want the Gini coefficient—and really, any measure of inequality—to obey this principle. It shows how money transfers (in the abstract) can reduce inequality, and we want our inequality measures to reflect that behavior.

(The fraction of wealth held by the top 10% is a measure which violates the Pigou–Dalton principle. For example, transferring money from one person to another who earns less when both are in the same decile does not change the inequality level.)

Here's something else useful about the Gini coefficient: If everyone's income were suddenly doubled, or multiplied by any positive number, inequality would stay the same. Smitha would still be earning five times as much money as Wilberforce. Wilberforce might be able to buy more stuff, but their relative positions haven't changed. Therefore, the inequality level should remain as is.

There are, unfortunately, limitations to the Gini. If everyone made $10 a year, the Gini coefficient would be zero—which is exactly the same inequality level if everyone made $1,000,000 a year. So the Gini doesn't give us useful information about actual incomes or wealth. That may seem like an obvious example, but it becomes important if you try to use it to compare inequalities across different countries.

In 2011, the Gini coefficient in the U.S. was 0.474, whereas in India, according to the World Bank, it was 0.351.[37, 159] This means that the U.S. has a higher level of inequality than India. However, the U.S. also has a higher per capita income and is richer, while India has a lower cost of living. There are other technical differences, such as how income is defined and counted in each country. Given this, it's difficult to make a meaningful comparison.

The Gini runs into similar ambiguities when you try to compare different regions within the same country. Figure 3.8 shows a graph of the 2017 inequality levels across the fifty states.[44] Utah has the lowest Gini coefficient at 0.4225, and New York has the highest at 0.5157. This gap between the Beehive State and the Empire State is quite large.

As both estimates were calculated using the ACS, we avoid the terminology problem ("What is income?") we had when comparing the U.S. to India. However, the issue of disparate living conditions remains. In 2017, around 3.1 million people lived in Utah, thinly spread over 82 thousand square miles. New York, however, had over 19.8 million residents, and is home to the twinkling, busy, maddening New York City, America's largest city.[33, 43] These are *very* different places in which to live and work.

There's one final property to consider: decomposability. (It's less gruesome than it sounds.) Look at that vertical line in Figure 3.8—it shows the Gini coefficient for the entire country. It was generated using the same household-level data that was used for

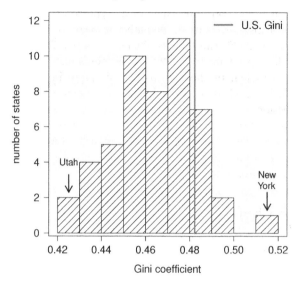

Figure 3.8 Gini coefficient distribution across states in the U.S. The vertical line represents the national inequality estimate for 2017. (Source: 2017 American Community Survey 1-year estimates.)

the state estimates. If the state estimates could be combined in some way to equal the national one without having to use the underlying household data, then a measure is decomposable.

The Gini coefficient, unfortunately, is not a decomposable inequality measure. There are other inequality measures out there, and many of them are decomposable such as the Thiel and Atkinson indices, and while they merit long discussions, we won't get into them here. That said, the Gini coefficient remains the most popular. Ultimately, the Gini coefficient (like all inequality measures) can tell us the level of inequality, but only we can determine whether that level is preferable, reasonable, or exploitative.

SUMMARY

Economists have devised a range of ways to measure and study inequality. The Gini coefficient, a single number between 0 and 1, is the most popular. CEO pay ratio, while striking, is not useful for official purposes and the top 1% (or top 10%) ignores most of the population; however, both are easy for a layperson to understand. Whichever measure is used, inequality appears to be worsening this century. In 2006, the Gini coefficient was 0.447 in the U.S.; by 2017, it had crept up to 0.482.[37] This seems like a small shift. But don't be fooled: In the real-world, this jump in the Gini coefficient can be tracked to the subprime mortgage crisis and the Great Recession.

Some inequality is expected due to differences in education, work ethic, experience, and so on. However, a level at which large swathes of the population have difficulty affording basic necessities is, by any measure, unfair.

FURTHER READING

The Economics of Inequality by Thomas Piketty and translated by Arthur Goldhammer. Harvard University Press, 2015.

In this slim volume, Piketty takes a historical look at inequality and examines the forces of social and technological change which produced major shifts in inequality worldwide. He advocates using a ratio of the lowest wage you can have but still be in the top decile over the highest wage you can have but remain in the bottom decile (P90/P10) rather than the Gini coefficient because it is simpler to compute. For a comprehensive, technical treatment of this subject, read Piketty's *Capital in the Twenty-First Century*.[125]

"The 1 percent's problem" by Joseph E. Stiglitz and Linda J. Bilmes. *Vanity Fair*, May 31, 2012.

This essay notes that inequality in the U.S. is widening, largely due to policy decisions which increased capital gains. They argue that it actually is in the top 1%'s best interest to care about the other 99%. Reasons include spurring demand, motivating workers, and engendering trust in democratic and economic systems. They reason that to preserve (and increase) their wealth, the "selfish solution" for the top is to promote a fairer system for all.

What Money Can't Buy: The Moral Limits of Markets by Michael J. Sandel. Farrar, Straus and Giroux, 2012.

This book takes us farther afield, but is a good companion to the article above. The standard economic view is that we "vote with our dollars." That is, if an item is worth more to us, we will pay a higher price for that product, shuffling our money away from items we value less to those we value more. Sandel asserts that this may be acceptable for things like yachts and upscale hotels, but the same principle should not apply to basic necessities such as food, housing, and healthcare. He notes that inequality is worsened by the idea that everything should be subject to market forces and that just because some things *can* be for sale does not imply that they *should* be.

CHAPTER 4

Housing

I N 1835, ADOLPHE QUETELET, best known for inventing the body mass index, published a lengthy treatise on the "Average Man." He cast his mold from measurements taken from 26,000 American soldiers, tabulating the average height, chest circumference, grip strength, and so forth.[150] Quetelet wanted to describe the "typical" male.

With the dimensions of Average Man, you could build all sorts of things. For instance, in 1926, the U.S. military began to construct cockpits based on the size of an average pilot. Sadly, a senseless number of planes built fitting these specifications crashed during non-combat flights.

Decades later, a lieutenant pointed out that (surprise!) no one actually looked like the average pilot. The cockpits had been designed so nobody could work properly in one. He suggested changing them to fit actual people. The accidents promptly ceased.[131]

Keeping that story in mind, picture the following:

New construction in leafy neighborhood with 3 bedrooms and 1.5 baths. Large yard, central air, and two car garage. Asking price $350,000.

Gorgeous Victorian built in 1897 with period features. Bring your contractor! 5 bedrooms and 3 baths. Within walking distance to town center and train station. Asking price $500,000.

Two bedroom, 2 bath apartment on 20ᵗʰ floor with ocean view. Large bedrooms and eat-in gourmet kitchen. Asking price $400,000.

Hyperbole and craftiness aside, how would you compare these three properties? It is hard to envision a "typical" house apart from the Hollywood version of a suburban home complete with a white picket fence and mischievous dog. And even this hypothetical house wouldn't necessarily have the average number of windows or bedrooms or yard size.

Average Man had these problems too. We could speculate whether it was reasonable to expect a man of average height to also have average chest circumference. Just like Quetelet's Average Man and the military cockpits, it is foolhardy to study housing thinking about an "average house." Rather, any analysis needs to account for the heterogeneity across homes.

Housing is an important part of an economy. Moreover, everyone needs a place to live so monitoring the state of a heterogenous housing market is a valuable activity.

Building permits are one way to track the housing market. Since developers only start to build a home if they feel they can sell it later, building permits are considered leading indicators about the economy.

House price indices are another measure of the housing market. S&P CoreLogic Case–Shiller Home Price Indices and the Zillow Home Value Index are two commercial examples. The Federal Housing and Finance Agency (FHFA) produces, among others, the House Price Index. This regulatory agency monitors organizations such as Fannie Mae and Freddie Mac.[70]

Below is a general categorization of house price index methods:

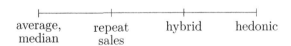

On the left side of the diagram are the simplest indices, average price or median price. They require only the time of sale and the price to be calculated. On the right are hedonic indices, the most complex. These can require lots of—possibly hard to find—information even if the calculations aren't too difficult.

Repeat sales indices look at how the price of a house changes each time it is sold. Finally, hybrid indices try to combine bits of repeat sales and hedonic. Median and repeat sales indices are the most popular types and so we will focus on them.

CALIFORNIA, HERE WE COME

Imagine you are moving to sunny San Diego, California. You need a place to live! As any realtor will tell you, it's all about location. We can learn about San Diego, the location, using the American Housing Survey (AHS).[57]

The AHS is a longitudinal survey conducted by the Census Bureau on behalf of the Department of Housing and Urban Development (HUD). HUD, which is part of the cabinet, uses the survey to develop its policies. It has existed in some shape or form since 1973. The "longitudinal" part just means that the occupants of the same house are interviewed across multiple years even if the residents themselves have changed.

Lots of information is collected in this survey from whether a house has air conditioning to the number of bedrooms to its proximity to a grocery store. This data is published at various geographic levels, including Core Based Statistical Areas (CBSAs). These are useful, but not official, regions that can be thought of as commuter zones around cities. They are defined by the Office of Management and Budget (OMB), part of the President's Executive Office.

For example, the CBSA containing New York City encompasses Long Island and northern New Jersey, even though the latter is an entirely different state. Larger CBSAs are called Metropolitan Statistical Areas and smaller ones are, not surprisingly, called Micropolitan Statistical Areas.[114]

San Diego is part of the San Diego–Carlsbad–San Marcos Metropolitan Area, which is outlined in the map of California in Figure 4.1 on page 54. Here, both macro and micro areas are identified and we can locate San Diego in a metro area which borders the Pacific Ocean and Mexico.[35] To make things simpler, whenever we say "San Diego" assume we are talking about its CBSA.

San Diego was part of the 2011 AHS when there were nearly 1.2 million homes in and around the city. These properties housed more than 3.1 million people.[57] (People living in more transient facilities such as college dorms were not included in this total.)

Looking at Table 4.2, we find that more than 60% of the 1.2 million residences in San Diego were attached homes, which do not have a yard on all sides, and detached homes which do. Both are considered single-family homes as opposed to apartments or mobile homes. As most indices are designed for single-family homes, we will focus on them in this chapter.

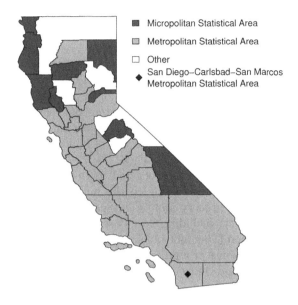

Figure 4.1 Map of California with CBSAs delineated. Metropolitan areas are shown in light gray and micropolitan areas in dark gray. The blank spots are regions which are not part of any major population center. San Diego is located in southwest California (diamond). (Source: Census Bureau, Geography Division.)

Let's circle back to your home search. Of the many homes in the city, only some will be for sale. Swirling among the myriad decisions you must make, there is ultimately one number which determines where you live: price. So, exactly how expensive *is* San Diego real estate?

Presumably, the price you pay for a home incorporates information about its size, the neighborhood, and even the rain showers in the bathrooms. On an aggregate level, a house price index tries to do something similar, but across many homes.

These indices are billed as representing the "housing market" but...(1) we are excluding nearly 40% of properties by focusing

TABLE 4.2   Types of homes within the area encompassing San Diego, Carlsbad, and San Marcos in California. (Numbers do not add up to total due to rounding.)(Source: 2011 American Housing Survey.)

units in structure	no. of homes (in thousands)
1, detached	621.6
1, attached	112.0
between 2 and 4	88.7
between 5 and 9	106.8
between 10 and 19	95.6
between 20 and 49	57.6
50 or more	61.3
manufactured/mobile home or trailer	42.7
total homes	1,186.1

only on single-family homes and ignoring apartments and mobile homes, (2) by looking at sales, we ignore the rental market, and (3) (most of the time) we learn nothing about the property values of homes in which people are currently living, only those which are sold.

The first two can be dispensed with by saying that house price indices only describe single-family home sales and nothing more. The third tells us that we really know little about a city, since so few homes are sold at any given time. For example, out of 733,600 single-family homes, only around 20,700—roughly 2.8%—were sold in 2011 in San Diego.[57, 151]

While sale prices of homes are part of the public record in the U.S., those records are scattered across local agencies countrywide. In the past, aggregating prices from each agency was slow and time-consuming. On the other hand, in the United Kingdom, the HM Land Registry, a government agency, compiles all home sales in one central location. With the advent of the internet and more efficient database tools, however, home sales can be collated more easily.

BASIC PRICE INDICES

To have any inkling of whether prices are increasing or decreasing, we at least need to know when houses are sold, at what price, and where they are located. If this is all we have, a reasonable place to start is to compute the average price, say, per month in San Diego.

The black line in Figure 4.3A shows just that for San Diego home sales between April 1995 through December 2013. From the graph, we can see the average price of a home steadily rise as we inch toward 2007, when the housing bubble really burst. And then, it plummets.

The average price gives us a feel for the direction house prices are taking, but can make the landscape look rosier than perhaps it actually is. Just like with people's salaries, home prices vary a lot and there are always a few mansions sold (or a few high earners) which bring up the average. Median sale price is consequently a more helpful measure. (The National Association of Realtors publishes a median sale price series as a general measure of the housing market.)

Like the median of a highway, the median sale price represents the middle price—50% of homes had a higher price, 50% of homes had a lower price. Therefore, a few expensive homes would not substantially alter the median price.

The blue line in Figure 4.3A is the median price for each month. The trend of the line is similar to the average price, but is shifted downwards. Furthermore, we can see that the median price line is less choppy. This is an example of how a few expensive homes sold throughout the year can make it look like San Diego house prices jump around a lot more than is the case.

This may be obvious, but using the median price has, well, price as its unit of measurement. Comparing across months is easy because we would just look at the difference in median (or average) prices. However, as we will soon discover, there are a number of ways to create indices which use the sale price for calculations but do not generate an index where price is the final unit of measurement.

On the surface, this seems like we are making things unnecessarily complicated. Prices are easy to interpret; perhaps we should retain that advantage. Another look at our average vs. median price graphs can give us a more nuanced view, however.

From Figure 4.3A, we can say that in any given month, average price is higher than median price. OK. That's a start. Can we say that average price is growing faster than median price? This is much harder because not only do we have to see how quickly a given series changed, we also have to compare the size of the gap between the two lines.

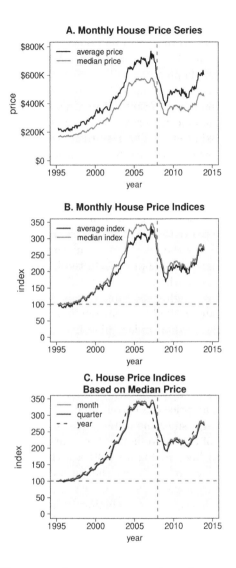

A. Monthly House Price Series

B. Monthly House Price Indices

C. House Price Indices Based on Median Price

Figure 4.3 These graphs compare various house price indices for San Diego using average and median sale prices. The vertical, dotted lines indicate the start of the Great Recession in December 2007. The base year where the index equals 100 is April 1995, marked by the horizontal line in graphs B and C. (Sources: Courtesy of Valuation Technology Inc.; National Bureau of Economic Research.)

This question would be far easier to answer if, in the first quarter, both series started at the same point. Then we could watch the two lines (possibly) diverge over time. A quick mathematical trick can make that happen.

In April 1995, the first month in our data, the average sale price was approximately $228,000. If we divide each average price (including the first month's price) by this initial value, we would get an index starting at 1. The resulting values are called price relatives. They convey the price in a given month *relative* to the price in April 1995. Similarly, the median price in April 1995 was around $167,000. If we repeat our trick, this index will start at 1 as well. We can then finish things off by multiplying everything by 100. This shifts the starting point from 1 to 100 for convention's sake. Now we are ready to do our comparisons.

Figure 4.3B shows the effects of calculating price relatives for our average and median sale prices. On the left at April 1995, we can see that the two methods have identical starting points at 100. Both indices follow roughly the same trends. We could see this to some degree in our original version, but it is simpler to confirm here. However, the median index (blue line) shows a higher rate of increase than the average index (black line) before the Great Recession started in 2007.

The choice between average and median indices mirrors the choice between using average or median wage in the inequality chapter. The median price is a better indicator of the housing market than the average, since the latter value can be affected by the sale of a handful of expensive homes (i.e., outliers).

However, both lines in Figure 4.3B are choppy. The primary reason is because we are splitting the sales data into groups by month and there are fewer sales per month than per quarter (combining three months) or year (combining 12 months). To be more specific, from 1995 through 2013, roughly 1,700 homes were sold on average per month; 5,200 each quarter; and 20,500 each year. The more sales information we have, the more stable our series will be from one time period to the next, which results in a smoother curve.

We can see this in Figure 4.3C as we move from month (blue line) to quarter (black) to year (dotted line). The downside of using long periods is that we have to sit around and twiddle our thumbs for a while before we can compute the next index value. By that time, our calculation may be outdated. Here, we will stick to quarters as a happy medium between months and years. (Many commercial indices also use quarters.)

ISN'T MEDIAN PRICE ENOUGH?

Some things differ from one quarter to the next which aren't immediately apparent from our graphs. Suppose you have children. If you can help it, you probably want to avoid moving in the middle of the school year. If lots of people have the same idea, we would expect to see more sales during the summer months. This type of pattern is called seasonality. (The labor force participation rate, from the jobs chapter in Figure 2.1A on page 9, also showed seasonal patterns.)

We can see this cyclical structure for San Diego in Figure 4.4 where the number of sales is graphed for each quarter. The regularity of the spikes shows seasonality. The peaks generally correspond to the summer months (triangles and squares) whereas the troughs (× symbols) are during the fall semester.

If school schedules are important to you, then school districts, playgrounds, and parks may be important to you too. Younger families—those who find these things important—tend to have less money at their disposal, since they have had a shorter time to accumulate it. This generally means they can only buy cheaper homes.

Another wrinkle emerges when we try to compare new homes with older ones. We want to know whether new homes are more expensive because of location or whether higher quality materials are used, for example.

Now we have a dilemma. Not only is there a difference in how many homes are sold each quarter, but there could be a difference in what kind of homes are sold as well.

Indices are supposed to help us figure out if housing is getting more or less expensive relative to previous quarters. However, these issues seem to muddle things even more. (The answer also depends on inflation which, curiously enough, is ignored in most house price indices.)

Essentially, we want to be sure that a rise in the index is because housing has actually gotten more expensive, not just because kids are on summer vacation or because a developer is installing marble countertops instead of granite ones. These questions are impossible to answer from a median or average price index.[107]

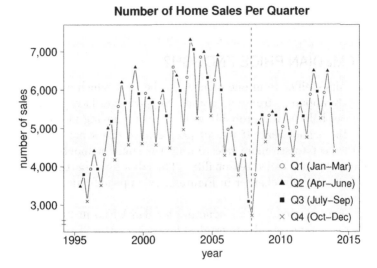

Number of Home Sales Per Quarter

Figure 4.4 This plot shows the seasonal (cyclical) pattern in the number of sales per quarter in San Diego. We can see the large drop in sales as we reach the Great Recession which began in December 2007. (Sources: Courtesy of Valuation Technology Inc.; National Bureau of Economic Research.)

BEDS, BATHS, AND A LOT MORE

Beyond price considerations, choosing where to live also has a uniquely personal side. Perhaps you are afraid of heights and avoid skyscrapers despite the striking scenery. Or maybe you like old homes with attics, cupboards under the stairs, and clawfoot tubs. Whatever your tastes, someone, somewhere likes the opposite.

However, what if we were able to say that an ocean view, on average, seems to raise the price of a home or that kitchens from the 1980s, on average, do the opposite. Hedonic indices are an attempt to quantify these types of characteristics. (Here, "hedonic" stands for attributes of a house, not hedonism.)

Perhaps we can figure out a way to determine how much each additional bedroom is related to the sale price. So far, this seems like a good idea. Our house price index could then be constructed after subtracting the effects of this hedonic information. This would mean we would make the following tradeoff: Use a more complicated method, but eliminate some of the problems which arise with median price indices.

Unfortunately, this brings up increasingly convoluted issues about what characteristics of a house we should include in the index. Bedrooms, bathrooms, square footage, and lot size seem like obvious ones to include. Others could be: distance to the city center, parks, or transportation links; views of an ocean, lake, or a brick wall; features like a jacuzzi, swimming pool, or air conditioning. And...this list could go on forever.

The stuff listed above is straightforward, although time-consuming, to ascertain. We can physically check if there is a pool or a working dishwasher. It is more difficult to determine exactly how good the view is or whether Brutalist architecture is currently in vogue. It is even harder to measure how well a house has been maintained.

We can make matters worse. First, the importance of various characteristics differs across cities. Basements are useful in tornado zones, but can be lethal in earthquake-prone regions. Second, some of these features could become more or less important over time. Open kitchens and intercoms are two such fads. This brings us to the third, most critical, problem: This is an impractical method.

For example, in our San Diego data, we have limited information on each house, like construction year and square footage, shown in Figure 4.5. As expected, there is a lot of variation across homes. Some are spacious, others are old, and many are both. But, these graphs are possible only because at some point in time, people collected this data for each and every house. And if any renovations were done, someone would have to update that data. This is a time- and labor-intensive exercise.

It is generally too difficult to make sure you know what the relevant characteristics are for each city, to be able to collect that data for each house, and to update that information whenever those attributes change. While the hedonic approach was the initial way people thought to construct a house price index, it was quickly abandoned because it caused far more problems than it solved.

ANOTHER SALE, ANOTHER PRICE

The downside of hedonic indices is that we need to amass a large amount of hedonic information before doing any calculations. This is nearly an impossible task to do well consistently over a long

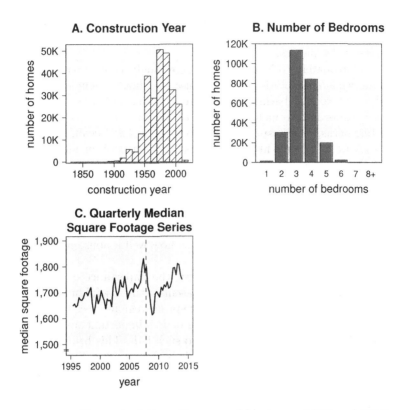

Figure 4.5 Characteristics of homes sold between 1995 and 2013 in San Diego. There is a steep drop in the median square footage of homes sold after the Great Recession began (dotted line) in plot C. (Sources: Courtesy of Valuation Technology Inc.; National Bureau of Economic Research.)

period of time and over a large geographic area. (That said, crowd-sourcing and web-scraping applications do make this more feasible.)

Instead, suppose after a long search, your offer on a lovely three-bedroom, two-bath home for $150,000 is accepted. Checking online records, you find that the seller purchased it for $100,000 ten years ago. Ignoring inflation, the price of this house rose $50,000 in the intervening decade.

In 1963, academics Martin Bailey, Richard Muth, and Hugh Nourse proposed that this $50,000 difference could be used to construct an index. The importance of the three bedrooms, the two bathrooms, or any other features would be irrelevant since we would be comparing the house with itself.

The two sales of the same house are called sale pairs. By averaging the price differences over many such sale pairs, they extracted the index value for each quarter. This type of approach is called a repeat sales index because it uses *repeat sales* of the same house.[10]

Instead of using sale prices directly, the researchers rescaled the prices first before computing their index. Before going ahead any further, let's take a slight detour to understand why.

In 1989, San Francisco was jolted by an earthquake of magnitude 6.9 on the Richter Scale. In 2017, Papua New Guinea suffered an earthquake of magnitude 7.9.[58] Both were powerful earthquakes causing fatalities and property damage.

As 7.9 is larger than 6.9, it stands to reason that Papua New Guinea had a more violent earthquake. However, based on the Richter Scale, a 7.9 earthquake is not slightly more powerful than one at 6.9, but *ten* times more powerful.

The Richter Scale was developed by academic Charles Richter in the 1930s. It is a logarithmic scale with base 10: Each additional unit on the scale results in a tenfold increase (i.e., a base-fold increase) in the severity of the tremors. This makes the scale more compact so magnitudes are not shooting off into the hundreds when violent earthquakes hit.

Similarly, logarithms make housing prices more compact by blunting the outliers. We can see this in Figure 4.6 by comparing graphs A and B. In A, we have our original prices. When there are a few very expensive houses—when our distribution is skewed right—we know that averages don't work well. This is important because the repeat sales method uses a statistical technique called regression, which is based on a certain kind of average.

Now, let's look at the graph in B. These are the same prices in the top graph but rescaled using the natural logarithm. (This means that the base is not 10, but e which is around 2.718. The mathematical constant e shows up in many places, including when calculating compound interest.) The shape of this graph is more symmetric, which is better when dealing with averages.

Our academic trio, Bailey, Muth, and Nourse, used these rescaled prices for their index. In effect, they said the difference in the rescaled prices of a sale pair was approximately equal to the difference in the rescaled index values at the time points that

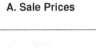

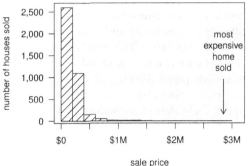

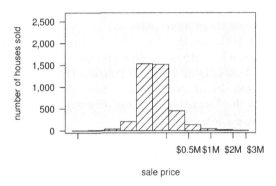

Figure 4.6 Graph A shows the distribution of all sale prices in a single quarter. Most houses sold for under $1 million, but a few went for much higher prices. In B, these prices are rescaled using a natural logarithmic transformation. Now the graph of rescaled prices shows a more symmetric shape, rather than the skewed shape in A. By labeling the horizontal axis in both A and B as sale price, we can see the effect of the transformation. Prices above $1 million—outliers—are made more compact, reducing the asymmetry in the data while retaining the rank order of sale prices. Rescaled prices are used in many repeat sales house price indices. (Source: Courtesy of Valuation Technology Inc.)

house was sold. They used regression to average prices over many sale pairs to obtain those house price index values.

So, let's think about this for a minute. You just bought your house. The index value for *this* quarter will depend not only on the $150,000 you just paid, but also the sale price the *last* time that house was sold. Both prices are used. One thorny issue we had with median (and average) price indices was that we couldn't control for different types of houses being sold in different quarters. Sharing information across quarters reduces that problem. One point for repeat sales indices!

For a long time, this method went unnoticed. In 1987, Karl E. Case and Robert J. Shiller relaunched it with a useful twist. (This is the same Shiller who won the economics Nobel Prize in 2013 for his work on asset prices.)

Now, say the house you just purchased for $150,000 sold for $100,000 not a decade ago but rather two decades ago. How would this change your opinion of the housing market?

In the first case, it took ten years for the price to increase by $50,000; in the second, it took double that. The original repeat sales index would simply swap the quarter of the previous sale with the older date, and continue along merrily.

However, a lot can happen in ten years. Supermarkets open. Recessions occur. Neighborhoods change. Our twenty-year-old price can feel rustier than the ten-year-old one.

Case and Shiller would agree with you. In Figure 4.7, we can see how much time elapses between sales in San Diego. Around 60% of people seem to move after living in their homes for at most five years (left side of graph), but there are a few who move after a few decades (right side). We, again, see a skewed shape.

It would be great to work these gap times into our index. Case and Shiller did so by adding a weight to each sale pair when computing the repeat sales index. Sale pairs with shorter gap times between sales were given more importance—that is, a higher weight— than those with longer ones.

As with all measures, there are some downsides to this approach. A quick look at Table 4.8 shows us one disadvantage. We know there are around 733,000 single-family homes in San Diego. Over the course of nearly 20 years some of these homes were put up for sale, a few more than once.

A lot of homes never went up for sale between 1995 and 2013 so they never show up in a repeat sales index. Of those that were sold, around 152,000 sold only once. These wouldn't show up in

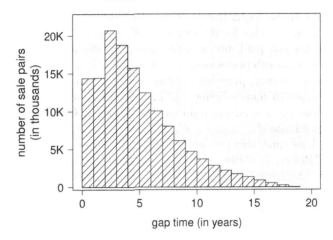

Figure 4.7 This histogram shows how much time elapsed between two sales of the same house across our San Diego data. Around 60% of resales occurred within five years of the previous sale. (Source: Courtesy of Valuation Technology Inc.)

our repeat sales index either. Only those homes which sold two or more times make up the "repeat" part of the repeat sales index. This subset comprises only 40% of the homes which were sold at some point between 1995 and 2013.

Excluding over half of home sales could be tolerable if the homes which sold multiple times were similar to those which did not. There is some evidence that this might not be the case. Moreover, we would have to completely forget about new homes until they sold a second time. Only then would they pop up in our sale pairs. This could be an issue for fast growing cities where lots of new houses are being built.

Among older homes, refurbishing or adding bathrooms could increase its price. Deterioration due to age could depress it. Or a house could get so old that it's deemed historic and command a higher price, like Victorians with gingerbread house trim.

Any of these changes—deliberate or otherwise—can occur. This means that we aren't really comparing the same house twice. There have been some indices which try to incorporate some of these

TABLE 4.8 This table shows the number of times each home in San Diego was sold between 1995 and 2013. Among those homes which were sold, the majority sold only once. (Numbers are rounded in the table.) (Source: Courtesy of Valuation Technology Inc.)

sales	0	1	2	3	4	more than 4
homes	a lot!	152,000	68,000	24,000	5,900	1,300

issues into the repeat sales setup.[107] An example is the repeat sales index published by the Federal Housing and Finance Agency (FHFA), which applies an adjustment for the age of the house. Let's see what this index looks like next, along with two commercial ones.

INDICES IN THE WILD

The FHFA's House Price Index and S&P CoreLogic Case–Shiller Home Price Indices are two examples of repeat sales indices. Both are based on Case and Shiller's technique. (However, Standard & Poor's do not rescale their prices before computing their index.[144])

Zillow, Inc. produces its own index called the Zillow Home Value Index. It is a median price index, but it's a bit different from the one we looked at earlier. Since not every house is sold each month, Zillow produces an estimate of what it would have sold at had it been on the market. They call this price a Zestimate® (Zestimate® is a trademark of Zillow, Inc.). It is considered to be the *value* of the house, not the price of a sale, and the method they use is proprietary. Their index is constructed by computing the median of the Zestimate® values each month.[164] (All three organizations produce multiple indices, but we will focus on those for single-family homes here.)

In Figure 4.9, we can compare these three indices for Chicago, Los Angeles, our current spot San Diego, and the U.S. capital, Washington D.C. In all four cities, we see that the general trends are similar across index methods although the FHFA index shows the largest discrepancy for Los Angeles and Washington, D.C.

The vertical line in each plot marks the start of the Great Recession in December 2007. (Lehman Brothers declared bankruptcy in September of 2008.) You can see the housing bubble burst in all four cities just before that recession, although Chicago's house prices declined the least.

Soon, headlines like these began sprouting: "Unlike stocks, home prices rarely collapse."[71] and "Survey cites four California

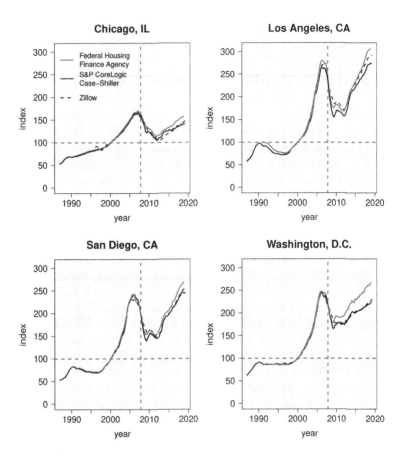

Figure 4.9 We compare the Federal Housing Finance Agency House Price Index (quarterly), S&P Core Logic Case–Shiller Home Price Index (monthly), and the Zillow Home Value Index (monthly). All indices have been seasonally adjusted; the indices have been rescaled so that they all equal 100 in March 2000. The vertical lines represent the start of the Great Recession in 2007. (Sources: Federal Housing Finance Agency; Courtesy of Standard & Poor's Financial Services LLC; Data provided by Zillow Group; National Bureau of Economic Research.)

banks with possibly risky realty loans."[11] People thought: How could this have happened? As it turns out, house prices have plunged before. Those headlines were written in the last century! Look back to Los Angeles. There is a smaller rise and fall around 1990. It looks small as the 2007 drop was far more dramatic, but this decline was painful too. Similar to subprime lending, banks were offering mortgages to those who had difficulty affording them.[107] History repeated itself in 2007. The house price indices show it.

SUMMARY

Comparing houses is tough whether you are a home buyer or a real estate agent. There are countless location, size, and amenity combinations. However, the goal of a house price index is to measure the "state of the housing market" which is itself a fuzzy concept.

One issue is that not all homes sell every quarter so many indices are based on limited sales information; others try to estimate what price a house may sell at using a statistical model or with an appraisal. Each approach we've discussed here—median price, hedonic, repeat sales—suggests a vastly different idea of what it means to quantify the state of the housing market. Despite these differences, however, they show similar overall trends.

In practice, it takes time for sales to be registered with local municipalities. Therefore, the index value for a given month is published several months later. Indices often have to be revised to incorporate sales which were registered very late. Often, adjustments are made after-the-fact to reduce seasonality as well (think school schedules), although they are not generally corrected for inflation.

FURTHER READING

Irrational Exuberance, Revised and Expanded Third Edition by Robert J. Shiller. Princeton University Press, 2015.

An earlier edition of this book was one of the first publications to note that the housing market was in a bubble before the 2007 housing and subsequent financial crisis. The third chapter of this book has an excellent history of housing and house price indices. Woven into this narrative, Shiller shows that contrary to popular opinion, housing is not necessarily *the* ideal investment. This is because house prices do not always increase once you adjust for inflation (the topic of our next chapter). The remainder of the book focuses on explaining how price bubbles are created, from systemic issues to the role of media.

Evicted: Poverty and Profit in the American City by Matthew Desmond. The Crown Publishing Group, 2016.

An engaging—but dispiriting—ethnography of both tenants and landlords who occupy the lower end of the rental housing market in Milwaukee, Wisconsin. Desmond deftly mixes in history and data to provide an aggregate picture about this often ignored and exploited segment of the population.

"When the (empty) apartment next door is owned by an oligarch," by Emily Badger. *The New York Times*, July 21, 2017.

Vancouver, London, Sydney, New York. These cities are increasingly drawing international home buyers. Homes bought are often left vacant, used as investment properties. From rising housing costs for city residents to businesses losing their customer base, this global trend has many local effects. The author describes this phenomenon and some ways governments are trying to address it.

CHAPTER 5

Prices

P EOPLE OFTEN CONVERT the fortunes of Gilded Age tycoons—
Rockefeller, Carnegie, Stanford—into current dollars to get a
sense of just how vast their fortunes really were. We could even
speculate about who was the richest person to have ever lived on
Earth.

BBC gives us as good a place to start as any: Musa I of Mali
(1280–1337), Zhao Xu (1048–1085) from China, or even Akbar I
(1542–1605) from India.[104]

Regardless of our internet search skills, it is impossible to answer this question. The obvious reason is an incomplete historical
record about who owned what. The second reason is we lack a lot
of information about how prices have changed over time. If we have
no concrete way of assessing the value of Musa I of Mali's posses-
sions in terms of today's currency, we cannot compare net worths
over the course of history.

The increase in prices across months (or years) is called inflation. (If prices decrease, it's technically called deflation.) In the
U.S., the Consumer Price Index (CPI) measures price levels and
inflation is measured by changes in the CPI. It has been computed
regularly since 1921, with calculations stretching back to 1913.[127]
Since then, we have been able to make more definitive judgments
about inflation.

The CPI is calculated by the Bureau of Labor Statistics (BLS),
the same division that publishes unemployment data. Also like unemployment, inflation is considered a lagging economic indicator.

For better or worse, the U.S. government has increasingly fix-
ated on inflation.[88] Salary increases are often calculated using these
price indices along with Social Security payments. The Federal

Reserve Bank sets monetary policy using another price index calculated by the Bureau of Economic Analysis (BEA) called the Personal Consumption Expenditures Price Index (PCE price index).

200 BANANAS SOLD TODAY, 500 TOMORROW

Let's say bananas cost 50 cents per pound last month and 60 cents
per pound today. If we divide these two numbers ($0.60/$0.50) =
1.2, we learn that bananas today are 20% more expensive than
they were last month. The 1.2 is called a price relative since we are
comparing the price today relative to the price last month. (We
also used price relatives in Figure 4.3B in the housing chapter.)

Figure 5.1 depicts these calculations for apple and banana
prices from January 1980 to October 2018.[18] The average monthly
price of apples and bananas per pound is graphed in plot A. We
can see that apples cost more per pound than bananas. However,
like with average house prices, this graph isn't good at establishing whether the price of apples grew faster or slower than that of
bananas. This is where price relatives are helpful.

If the fruit price each month is divided by its price in the first
month (January 1980), we get a string of price relatives. This pro-
cession of numbers is a rudimentary price index. January 1980 is
the base month of this index since we divided all the prices by the
price in that month. As the base month's price gets divided by
itself, the index value in January 1980 is 1. (Just like with house
price indices, we multiply everything by 100 so that the base period
value is 100 instead of 1.)

Our very own Apple and Banana Price Indices are plotted in
Figure 5.1B. We can see that apple prices fluctuate more than
banana prices. (Some of that volatility could be because of the
growing season for each fruit and having to import or refrigerate
fruit off-season.) We can also detect that prices for both fruits grew
at roughly the same pace until about 2000, at which point apple
prices started to grow at a faster rate than those for bananas.

This rate of growth is inflation. One way to extract it is to
calculate the percent change in the index from one month to the
next. Figure 5.1C shows those percent changes. For fruits, the line
is far more squiggly before 2000 than after. That tells us that prices
were more volatile, month to month, in the 1980s and 1990s.

We've gone from average price to price index to a crude inflation
measure, but we still don't know whether price movements were
demand-driven or supply-driven. For that, we need information not

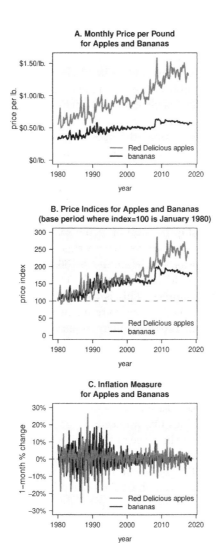

Figure 5.1 Average prices of apples and bananas (plot A) can be converted into a rudimentary price index (plot B) using price relatives. The percent difference in the index from month to month is a crude measure of inflation (plot C). (The official price indices for these two fruits use a slightly different formula.) (Source: Bureau of Labor Statistics.)

only on prices, but also on how many apples and bananas were sold each month. Let's see how quantities were gradually incorporated into price indices next.

Englishman Rice Vaughan outlined the first notion of a price index, which was published posthumously in 1675. At that time, wages for people like carpenters and servants were controlled by regulations that incorporated how much things like clothing and food cost. Vaughan compared wages and found prices had risen between 6 and 8 times over the past century.[46]

Bishop William Fleetwood, also from England, continued along these lines in 1707. At that time, students who earned more than £5 per year were ineligible for a fellowship at the University of Oxford. A student complained to Fleetwood that he was in danger of losing his fellowship because of a rule set in the 15th century.

It's almost too easy to see where this story is going. At the start of 2019, £5 was worth around $6.36. Based on our earlier calculations, this would buy us roughly 11 pounds of bananas or almost 5 pounds of apples. This is too little to feed even a small monkey for a year. The student's argument was that even in 1707, £5 per year was not nearly enough to survive. Fleetwood agreed and set about trying to show just that.

Fleetwood brought some key ideas to the development of price indices. To start, he selected a group of items: wheat, oats, beans, ale, cloth, beef, mutton, and bacon. (No veggies!) This was what we now call a market basket of goods. They were supposed to be representative of things Oxford students might buy.

He also compared the price of these goods at two time points—in the mid 1400s to his present—and computed price relatives, just like we did. Most of his goods had risen sixfold, the others fivefold.

His final step was to combine the price relatives into a combined index. He essentially averaged the price relatives to conclude that prices overall had risen nearly 6 times. What cost £5 back then would cost between £28 and £30 in 1707.[72] Therefore, Oxford's rule about fellowships was rather unfair.

And this is an ongoing point of debate: how to combine price relatives to produce a single index. Fleetwood decided to compute the average. (This is pretty much what Gian Rinaldo Carli, an Italian economist, proposed in 1764.[46]) However, earlier in his book, Fleetwood proposed another method, which is now called the fixed basket approach.[62]

Fleetwood's basket included 5 quarters of wheat (1 quarter = 8 bushels), 4 hogshead of beer (1 hogshead is around 64 U.S. gallons), and 6 yards of cloth.[72] He then suggested the total price of this group of items be computed for two different years, then and now. That way we would know how much it would cost to get the same amount of stuff for both periods. Finally, by taking the price relative of the two total costs (total cost now/total cost before), he would see if prices rose, fell, or stayed the same. That is, he would get his index value.

While he eventually ended up taking an average of the individual item price relatives, his fixed basket method is considered the first formula for price index calculations. It's called a fixed basket because the items and their quantities (5 quarters of wheat, etc.) are held constant over the two time periods.

The person credited with refining this method was a third Englishman, Joseph Lowe in 1823. He suggested different market baskets depending on whether you were a laborer, farmer, and so forth. He also pushed for governments to produce price indices or at least provide the data so that others could construct them.[62]

Eventually the fixed basket method caught on and a wide cast of characters developed their own formulas. One big question was how to incorporate the quantity of goods. Why 5 quarters of wheat and not 10? Why 6 yards of cloth instead of 4?

INDEX FORMULAS

Price indices have four common elements:

1. constituents of a market basket of goods and services,

2. weights of the constituents,

3. prices of the constituents,

4. and a method to combine weights and prices.

Let's say we wanted to create a "Fruit Price Index." The first step would be to establish the constituents of the market basket. We need to determine whether apples and bananas are sufficiently representative of all fruits. That means we would be ignoring oranges and grapes and strawberries. Whether or not this is a reasonable subset would depend on how large of a proportion apples and bananas are of all the fruit sold in the country. (Hint: It's not. The CPI includes many other fruits.)

For simplicity, we will continue using apples and bananas as our market basket. Next, we must assemble a history of prices and

TABLE 5.2 Imaginary Fruit Price Index components.

item	previous month price/lb.	quantity	current month price/lb.	quantity
banana	$1.50	50 lbs.	$1.80	60 lbs.
apple	$1.00	300 lbs.	$1.50	250 lbs.

quantities, as in Table 5.2. (These quantities would eventually be translated into weights.[17])

We have our market basket, two sets of prices, and two sets of quantities. Most economists thought quantity should be tethered to how much of each item was sold either today or last month (or year, etc.) when comparing prices. Here are some ways to do so, named after their inventors:

- Laspeyres index (fixed basket) $\longrightarrow$ use previous month's quantities,

- Paasche index (fixed basket) $\longrightarrow$ use current month's quantities, and

- Fisher's ideal index $\longrightarrow$ use the previous and current month's quantities as this index is a geometric mean of the Laspeyres and Paasche indices (see below for geometric mean discussion).

At this point we need to explain the difference between an arithmetic mean and a geometric mean. Most of us compute arithmetic means, or averages, frequently. We add up the n values and divide by the number of values, or n, to get our average. This exercise is popular with the student feverishly calculating his GPA, the researcher computing average income, or even you estimating your average credit card bill. What all these tasks have in common is they are comparing similar items—GPAs, income, and credit card expenditure.

There are two cases when this proves to be problematic. The first is if you want to repeat this task across different items—for example an average of credit card expenditure and annual income. Given that annual income is likely to be significantly larger than credit card expenditure, changes in income will dominate the calculation. The second is if you are working with percentages instead of raw values; using a geometric mean takes into account the effects of compounding—of which a typical example is returns on the stock market.

A geometric mean is just another kind of average. Instead of adding the values, we multiply them. Instead of dividing by n values, we take the nth root. For example, the arithmetic mean of 2 and 8 is 5, as $(2+8)/2=5$. The geometric mean, on the other hand, is 4 because we need to compute the square root of 2×8.

If the 2 and the 8 were converted to percentage increases of prices, for example, the geometric mean would be the appropriate type of mean to use. This is because it could account for the fact that the price changed by 2% and then by an additional 8% on top of that; that is, it could account for compounding. The arithmetic mean does not have this capability.

As it stands, it's unclear which index—Laspeyres, Paasche, or Fisher's ideal—is the best choice. If, however, we try to implement these indices in practice, two options quickly become untenable.

Paasche and Fisher's ideal price indices both need information about quantities sold in the present. This type of information can only be known *after* the time period is over and it takes a while to compile. Inflation measures need to be timely, not calculated at a leisurely pace. Therefore, both are out.

That leaves Laspeyres!

Early on, the Bureau of Labor Statistics (BLS) calculated the CPI using a version of the Laspeyres index. Slowly, however, people starting thinking fixed baskets weren't flexible enough to accommodate long-term trends. For instance, as things become more expensive, most people change their spending habits by substituting one product for another. A variable basket method would allow for such (realistic) substitutions. One version, which incorporates geometric means, is called the expenditure-share-weighted geometric mean index. We'll call this the EWGM index. BLS switched to this method in 1999.

The "expenditure-share-weighted" part of the EWGM is a way to set the importance of each product to the overall basket. These weights change as people adjust their spending on various goods for various reasons, including in response to changing prices. Another advantage of this type of price index is that it's a better approximation of a cost of living index (more on that at the end of this chapter).

The Laspeyres index, however, is still currently used for a few things, including rented housing, electricity and water, and physicians' services.[17] On the other hand, the PCE price index, uses a version of the Fisher's ideal index and a slightly different market basket of goods compared to the CPI.[15] (Because of these differences, the CPI and PCE price index do not yield the same index values.)

URBAN LIVES AND URBAN PRICES

Early reports on prices were ad hoc in the late 1800s. They were often used for one-off purposes and focused a lot on food prices. This mostly was due to a spotty budget for the Bureau of Labor (now BLS).

For instance, in September 1915, price relatives for only 17 foods were published, most of which were meat or dairy items (no apples and bananas yet).[26] By 1921, the list had expanded to 44 items (including bananas) with price relatives across 51 cities. Slowly, the categories became increasingly refined: sirloin steak, round steak, rib roast, chuck roast, plate beef; butter, oleo margarine, nut margarine, lard, crisco.[23]

Royal Meeker, the third commissioner of the Bureau of Labor, pressed for extensive surveys of family expenditures, income and expenditures of low-earning white women, and a study of dietary habits of families living in the District of Columbia. (Only non-governmental employees were included.) Part of his pitch to Congress was that he wanted to answer the question: "What does it cost the American family to live?" His plea worked and he received money to carry out the studies.

The data was collected at the start of 1917 and by the end of the year, he had some results. It turned out that things were quite dire. Most low-income families could not afford enough food; women were working for very little and for long periods of time, implying that they couldn't, therefore, be homemakers.[78]

A second push from Meeker came through a request from the Shipbuilding Labor Adjustment Board. By this time, the U.S. was in the midst of World War I (they entered in April of 1917). Prices were rising and wages needed to keep up. Therefore, price indices were needed to properly adjust those wages.[78]

In early 1918, Meeker received funding to study the families who lived and worked around shipyards in selected cities. For example, 104 families were interviewed in Portsmouth, New Hampshire. They spent, on average, $1,406.97 over a year. Nearly half of this amount was spent just on food. Food prices had risen around 47% in a little more than three years for this group; the cost of "Furniture and furnishings" had risen a staggering 84%. On the other hand, housing had only gone up by 3.28%. Overall, in Portsmouth, prices were deemed to have risen nearly 46%.[21] These tidbits let us sense the struggles Portsmouth families faced.

Apart from wartime needs, regular life in the U.S. shifted rapidly in cities bringing a need for regular information on prices. During the early 1900s, the way people shopped began to change. They started going to stores and buying more finished goods. Bargaining was on the decline. People began to grumble when prices rose as it was hard to go back to making your own stuff.

Lots of people thought this indicated that people were living beyond their means and being irresponsible. But, this wasn't really the root of the problem. There were a lot of issues, including "industrial collusion" which affected prices in ways which made things difficult for consumers.[145] This was why the need for price indices became more pressing.

Slowly, the number of cities surveyed started to expand beyond those with shipyards to more industrial cities. Price indices started to be published regularly in 1921.[127] The published tables became increasingly voluminous as well.

These initial price indices were called cost of living indices, although that was a bit of a misnomer. That term was eventually dropped in favor of the Consumer Price Index, or CPI.

There are two common threads throughout these initial attempts. First, they looked exclusively at cities, not rural areas. Second, they considered only wage workers (people who weren't salaried employees).

Currently, there are two main versions of price indices published by BLS: CPI-U and CPI-W. The "U" stands for urban and is intended to represent everyone who lives in cities, about 88% of the population.

While CPI-U is the one everyone talks about, the CPI-W is actually the older index. The "W" in CPI-W stands for households where at least 50% of household income comes from wages and clerical workers' earnings.[17] The "W" also only looks at urban areas and is a subset of the households considered in the CPI-U.

If we look back to Meeker's studies, only lower-income families were interviewed. Changes in price affected such households a lot. In the late 1880s and early 1900s, industry, government, and labor unions were frequently arguing and so labor policy was a prominent issue. Consequently, CPI-W was used frequently to arbitrate labor disputes between unions and firms.[129]

Figure 5.3A shows the monthly CPI-U calculated all the way back to 1913.[18] The base period is 1982–1984 where the CPI-U is

100. This choice is important since an index is calculated relative to its base year. (This was also the case with house price indices.)

If you choose a base year that is abnormal—like when there is famine or a war going on—price changes in other years are going to be magnified in comparison. This is because all subsequent index values are interpreted in relation to the (atypical) base period. Consequently, you want to choose a time period which is humdrum so price comparisons are meaningful.

If we look back to Figure 5.3A, the series looks like a steady upward chug with maybe a small blip around 1920. All we can really say is that prices have risen since 1913; that is, we see inflation.

This serene curve belies some pretty dramatic swings because the time covered is over one hundred years long. Instead, we should look at Figure 5.3B to interpret inflation trends.

On the horizontal axis, like in the first plot, we have year. On the vertical axis, however, we have the percent change from the previous year. That is, how much prices changed, in percentage terms, each month compared to the same month the year before. We are comparing price changes from July to the previous July instead of comparing July with June because the series is not seasonally adjusted. (Versions of the CPI exist which are seasonally adjusted.)

Inflation is technically when money is worth *less* whereas deflation is when it is worth, comparably, *more*. On this graph, parts of the graph which are above zero are, roughly speaking, times of inflation since prices rose and so a dollar was worth less. Deflationary periods approximately correspond to periods where the graph falls below zero.

As you can see from Figure 5.3B, inflation was quite high when the U.S. fought in World War I (April 1917–November 1918). The war brought with it price controls and rationing which made use of inflation measures, along with wage adjustments like we saw with the shipyards. Government funds allocated for measuring inflation increased during this period, only to fall after.

In the 1920s, inflation was less volatile. During this period Irving Fisher tried to push for his ideal index to be used. Others argued against it, pointing out that at least with a fixed basket, since the quantities didn't change, you could be sure that changes in the index were only due to changes in price. While, the Laspeyres index continued to be used, the index formula debate would continue to crop up from time to time.[129]

The next dramatic period was during the Great Depression which began in late 1929 and continued through the early 1930s.

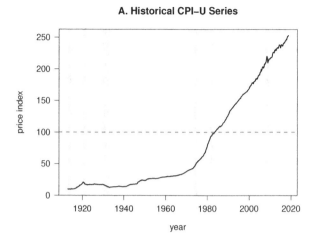

A. Historical CPI–U Series

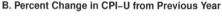

B. Percent Change in CPI–U from Previous Year

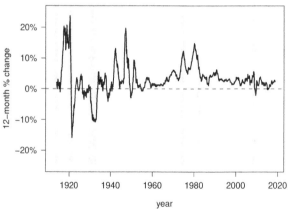

Figure 5.3 Plot A shows the monthly, U.S. City Average CPI-U calculated back to 1913. The base period is 1982–1984 and the series has not been seasonally adjusted. Plot B shows the percentage change between the CPI-U in one month and the CPI-U the same month in the previous year. The shaded areas represent the Great Depression and the major recessions in the U.S., including the 1973 and 1979 oil crises and the Great Recession. (Sources: Bureau of Labor Statistics; National Bureau of Economic Research.)

You can see this period in Figure 5.3B because most of the percent change values are below 0, that is, this is a deflationary period.

As we saw in the unemployment chapter, President Herbert Hoover didn't manage the crisis well and Franklin D. Roosevelt won the subsequent election in 1932. At that time the federal deficit was running high and large swathes of the population were living in misery.

Around two weeks after Roosevelt became president, Congress passed the Economy Act of 1933 with the goal of reducing the federal deficit. In addition to cutting veterans benefits, it also reduced federal employee salaries by 15%. The latter was justified by pointing to the fact that the country was in a deflationary period and therefore you needed less money to buy stuff.

Then Secretary of Labor, Frances Perkins, noted that the current method of measuring inflation (and deflation) was absurd. Thanks, in part, to a languishing budget, inflation was still calculated based on expenditure data from 1917–1919. As a result, things like household electricity were not yet being factored into the price index formulas. And so, in 1935, the federal government allotted funds to figure out how to update the methodology for measuring inflation.

Eventually, the U.S. formally entered World War II in December of 1941, bringing about another inflationary period. Here too, price controls and rationing were implemented. Inflation measure methodology had to be quickly updated to respond to these changes.

Gasoline rationing and bans on the production of various consumer goods meant that cars were eliminated from the index and public transportation received a higher weighting. Sometimes products were temporarily dropped because you couldn't actually find them at the store, like radios and metal bedsprings.[157] Inflation measures were also used to "cap wage increases" which brought some extra scrutiny to BLS.

Until this time, the inflation measure was called a cost of living index. Many people complained that the measure was underestimating inflation (the opposite complaint would become more common after World War II).

It was also pointed out that the cost of living index actually didn't live up to its name so BLS proposed "Consumer's Price Index for Moderate Income Families in Large Cities" instead. Perkins thought that was a terrible idea, saying, "The people who object to this index don't object to its name, you know." Eventually, after Perkins left her post, the new name was adopted in 1945.[78, 129] This index is what we now call CPI-W.

After World War II, which officially ended in September of 1945, the budget for the CPI slumped again, only to be refunded by Congress at the insistence of General Motors executives after some labor disputes.

In 1961, a commission, headed by George Stigler (who won the economics Nobel Prize in 1982), suggested shifting from the fixed basket idea to a "constant utility" idea. This way, new products and shifts in consumer spending could be incorporated into the index more naturally.

Their suggestions didn't take hold immediately. They resurfaced again in the mid 1990s with another commission, headed by Michael Boskin. The goal, now, was to shoot for a cost of living index. In practice, it would be approximated using a variable basket method and the EWGM formula. This was actually implemented in 1999 when the Laspeyres method was dropped for measuring price changes for most products and services. The Boskin Commission results also led to a third kind of inflation measure, the Chained CPI-U which was even closer to being a cost of living index in 2002 (more on that at the end of the chapter).[129]

Post-World War II, the idea of monitoring and ultimately controlling inflation became increasingly dominant. Roosevelt even referred to inflation as the "enemy."[129] Slowly, inflation was beginning to be used for many things beyond wartime. In fact, a third of federal expenditures had ties to the CPI by 1981.

All of this made politicians nervous that an uptick in inflation could mean higher payments for things like Social Security. The oil crises and "stagflation" of the 1970s didn't help either.

Also in the 1970s, President Richard Nixon started to require a measure of "core inflation" to be published. This was inflation minus food and energy (e.g., gasoline, electricity, natural gas) since they were considered more volatile, overshadowing what was, evidently, really going on (more on this later).[124]

President Gerald Ford even tried to get the public involved in fighting inflation by encouraging them to develop responsible spending habits through his Whip Inflation Now campaign. (His WIN campaign had some fetching paraphernalia including duffel bags and footballs.[127])

Since inflation was being used for more things, the government decided that it should be more representative of the U.S. population. So in 1974, during Ford's administration, BLS announced that the CPI-U would be making an entrance. This new measure would focus on everyone living in cities, and so represented a far larger percentage of the U.S. population.

By the time the CPI-U started being published alongside the CPI-W in 1978, Jimmy Carter was president. President Carter's administration also began to require the Federal Reserve Bank to manage inflation through monetary policy. People started to wonder whether speculating about future inflation ended up bringing about more inflation.[127]

So, everyone is worried about inflation and it's become a key indicator. Because of (or in spite of) that attention, the last 30 years or so has been a quieter period. (This is visible in Figure 5.3B because the squiggles are less intense than in the early 1900s.)

NEW IN AISLE 3: TV DINNERS

Along with apples and bananas, BLS collects prices on many goods and services including:

sandwich spreads	magazine subscriptions
distilled spirits at home	automobile service clubs
housekeeping services	rental of DVDs or video games
salt	sewing machines
food from vending machines	admissions to sporting events
wallpaper tools	pet food
fresh cut flowers	dental services
light bulbs	car or van pools
organ meats	delivery services
funeral services	credit card fees
decorative pillows	cigarettes
men's bathrobes	legal services
watches	gift wrap

These are extremely specific categories. For example, food that wasn't cooked at home is divided into: food eaten while in a sit-down restaurant, fast food, delivered meals, meals eaten at school or work cafeterias, vending machine purchases, food from mobile vendors, food at catered events, and so forth.

All of these minute categories are eventually combined to create the more than 200 individual components of the CPI called "items."[17] These items make up the, possibly familiar term, "market basket of goods."

Which items are on this list or not on this list—the market basket—is determined using the results from the Consumer Expenditure (CE) Survey. This is a combination of two surveys, the Interview and Diary Surveys, which ask people about their income and purchases. The data is collected by the Census Bureau on behalf of BLS.

"Consumer units" are contacted to participate in one of the two surveys. These units include families, but also include groups of people who live together and who make at least two of the following financial decisions together: housing, food, and living expenses.

The Interview Survey asks respondents what purchases they have made in the past few months, four times over the course of a year. It's easy to remember paying the electric bill or buying a new washing machine. It's harder to recall the chewing gum bought at the gas station or every vegetable purchased at the grocery store.

For that reason, this survey is supplemented with the Diary Survey. Here, the people in the selected consumer units must record every single thing they bought each day for two weeks.

Thousands of households participate in these surveys each year in urban areas across the country. The results are used: (a) to determine the market basket of goods and (b) to decide how important those goods and services should be when calculating the CPI. The latter are called weights and we will return to them in the next section.

The items in the market basket should reflect what people are buying. It's not surprising that apples are in the market basket. What is interesting, however, is that only Red Delicious apples are tracked. More apples of this type were eaten than any other in the U.S. until 2018 when it was overtaken by the Gala apple.[80] If the Red Delicious continues to lose its popularity, when (if at all) should it be replaced by another variety?

This question can go both ways in terms of deciding when to add items or when to remove or give them less importance. For example, high-button shoes were replaced by oxfords by 1935.[157] Silk slips were temporarily dropped during World War II because you could no longer buy them in stores; consequently, women replaced them with rayon slips, so their weight in the index was increased.[157] In 1951, frozen foods and televisions were added to the market basket of goods.[17]

Before combining everything in the market basket into a single index, the price index for each item is computed separately. This

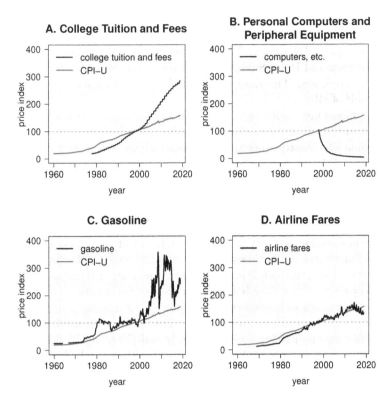

Figure 5.4 CPI-U (blue) with various item-level indices (black) from 1960 onward. These products and services are components of the CPI-U and CPI-W. The base period where the index is 100 is January 1998 for all indices; none of the indices have been seasonally adjusted. (Source: Bureau of Labor Statistics.)

is because prices can change more rapidly for some categories of items than others, and it's helpful to know those trends.

Figure 5.4 shows a few examples.[18] In each graph, the CPI-U is graphed along with a specific price index say, for instance, housing. By comparing the two lines, we can see whether item prices have been rising faster or slower than the overall index.

College tuition has risen much faster than the overall price index (i.e., CPI-U) in Figure 5.4A. In comparison, the relative price of a computer, shown in B, has plummeted. The trends for gasoline and airfare (graphs C and D) are mixed. Sometimes those prices grew faster, other times slower than the CPI-U.

In addition to these trends, we can see the lines for college tuition, gasoline, and airfare are choppier. The tiny zig-zag patterns for college tuition occur primarily because universities have cyclical schedules resulting in a seasonal effect. The airfare and gasoline indices have a bit of that too. Adjustments can be made to the data to better distinguish between changes in price due to season as opposed to an actual shift in the price. The result would be a smoother graph. However, even after such modifications, the graph for gasoline would still be choppy. This is simply because the price of gasoline is more volatile compared to something like college tuition.

Finally, out of the four items in Figure 5.4, only gasoline existed in 1960. College tuition, for example, was only added in the late 1970s.

People have been going to college for hundreds of years, but for most of that time, too few people attended to matter. Even in 1940, only 10% of people older than 25 had completed at least one year of college. By 1970, that number had risen to about 20%.[40] (These statistics are about the entire U.S., not just the urban populations considered in the CPI-U, for which we might expect slightly higher percentages.)

However, based on expenditure data, BLS decided in the 1970s that paying for college was a pervasive and important enough activity to add to the CPI. The same could probably be said about airfare, which became a category in the early 1960s.

The 200-odd items in the market basket aren't intended to represent a typical household. Not every family buys a new car, sends someone to college, and buys new bedroom furniture all in the same year, let alone the same month. Rather, the market basket is supposed to reflect what Americans buy in aggregate.

WEIGHTY MATTERS

As we just saw, the products and services from the CE Survey are combined to form more than 200 categories, called items. Prices for these items are collected from nearly 40 geographic areas all over the country. Some areas are obvious: New York, Chicago, Los Angeles. Some are distinctive: Anchorage, Honolulu. Others are groups of cities: the Midwest region includes Columbus and Dayton, Ohio, for example.

This gives us roughly 8,000 item-area combinations. Each of these has its own index. They aren't published because they contain too little data to be reliable. Instead they are merged in various arrangements.

CPI-U and CPI-W values are produced by aggregating all of the item-area indices. Item indices, on the other hand, combine indices for a given item across all geographic areas (like our apple and banana indices). Similarly, an area index merges all of the item-area indices for a particular city or region. There are also various other groupings of items and areas to get more category-specific indices, like food or energy indices.

In our own household budgets, we probably spend far less on toothpaste than on fruit. Chances are, we purchase more pounds of fruit than tubes of toothpaste too.

This means when combining item-area indices, they shouldn't be all treated equally. Weights are what specify how important each item and geographic area are to the final index. They must sum to 100 because all of the items comprise 100% of the market basket. (This is the "weighted" part of the EWGM method.)

The CE Survey is used to determine the weights. They are based on the total amount spent on a good or service in a given year in a particular geographic area. These weights change over time as economies shift, making the CPI a variable basket index.

Some of the shifts in spending patterns, for example, come from people who decide that maintaining a car is too expensive and switch to public transport. This is a change in spending across item categories, requiring the weights to be revised.

On the other hand, whether they be skinny jeans or bell bottoms, pants are simply pants as far as the BLS is concerned. Changing preferences within a category does not matter unless people start spending more within that category.

The story changes, however with all things tech-related. Technological advances bring new types of products to the CPI. New items require all of the weights to be re-jiggered, since the weights must add up to 100.

We saw in Figure 5.4B that personal computers (and peripheral equipment) became their own item in the market basket in the late 1990s. This was not the year PCs were invented. The first personal computer, the Altair, arrived on the scene in 1974.[66] Rather, like college tuition, it was added when it became an important enough spending category in the CE Survey.

CPI–U Weights

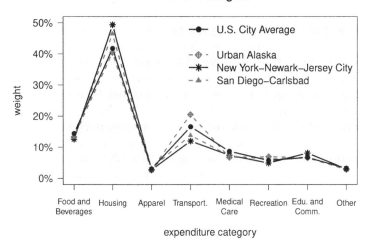

Figure 5.5 Relative importance of the eight major categories of products and services in the CPI-U for various geographic areas. Weights across expenditure categories sum to 100%. (Source: Bureau of Labor Statistics, 2015–2016 weights used for 2017 indices.)

Weights differ across items, but they also differ across geographic regions, or areas. (Remember, the basic price indices are item-area combinations.) Figure 5.5 gives us a sense of the regional differences across weights.[22] Here, the various items have been grouped to form the eight categories listed in the horizontal axis. The weights on the vertical axis are the sum of the weights of the items within each of those categories.

The line for the U.S. city average corresponds to the weights in the CPI-U. Since it integrates the indices for all items and all areas, the other lines on this graph are incorporated within this one.

Among the regions shown in the figure, the New York metropolitan area has the highest weight for housing, whereas Urban Alaska—with data from Anchorage—has the lowest. Housing also has the distinction for being the highest weighted category, accounting for more than 50% of expenditures. (The physical residence, "shelter," and the things you need to furnish and run it are all part of housing.)

The reverse pattern is true for transportation: Urban Alaska is now the highest and New York City, with an extensive public transportation system, is the lowest. Both transport and food are weighted roughly between 10 and 20%.

The San Diego area, for which we examined house price indices, is somewhere in the middle for all eight categories.

Given that it takes time for data to be collected and processed, weights are computed using older, not current CE Survey data. The implicit assumption is that consumer spending patterns aren't changing a lot within a short time span, so using old weights won't make much of a difference. This didn't end up being quite the case, so adjustments are made to correct for that.[129]

Now that we've looked at the composition of the market basket and the weights, we can finally turn to pricing.

AND THE PRICE IS...

Imagine you receive a phone call from the Census Bureau. They want to know whether you've purchased any of the following:

new motorcycles $\longrightarrow$ within 5 years
sewing machines, fabric, or sewing supplies $\longrightarrow$ within 1 year
intracity mass transit $\longrightarrow$ within 3 months
parking fees or tolls $\longrightarrow$ within 1 month
canned fruits or vegetables $\longrightarrow$ within 2 weeks
gasoline, diesel, or alternative fuels $\longrightarrow$ within 2 weeks

Along with each category, there is a time span to help jog your memory. When you bought an expensive, infrequent purchase like a motorcycle is easy to remember, hence the 5-year period. Things you buy more regularly, like gasoline for that motorcycle, have a shorter time span. It's simpler to remember where and when you bought gas last week, as opposed to last month.

Let's say you tell the Census Bureau employee you bought applesauce yesterday, which falls under the "canned fruits or vegetables" category. You tell them how much you paid and that you bought it at your local grocery store. The interview ends, and you hang up.

This interview is part of the Telephone Point of Purchase Survey (TPOPS). It's administered by the Census Bureau on behalf of BLS. The people selected to participate are contacted four times over the course of a year and asked about some of their purchases.

The goal of TPOPS is to assemble and update a list of retail outlets on where people shop.

The next step in the process is called the Commodities and Services sample (C&S sample). Stores are selected from the list of outlets curated from TPOPS. Each store is then assigned a set of products. Someone with the job title Economic Assistant visits the stores and records prices for the specified products. The CPI is calculated using those prices.

Thanks to your hot tip about applesauce, your local grocery store was chosen to be part of the C&S sample. Say Frank, the Economic Assistant, sets out looking for applesauce. A bewildering array of options awaits. There are regular and organic applesauces. There are difference sizes. Some have sugar, some artificial sweeteners. And there are many, many brands.

Frank has a strategy to whittle these options down to a single product, say Applesauce W. He records the price. He then moves on to the other items on his list, Butter X, Pasta Y, and Soup Z. For the next few years, he continues visiting the same store and recording prices for the exact same items.

One day, Frank visits the retail outlet and finds that Applesauce W is no longer available. Here too he has a procedure to substitute a similar product along with a method to account for the difference in quality. (This happens all the time for apparel pricing since seasons change and so does what's in style.)

To give some sense of scale of the C&S sample, prices for around 83,400 products and services are collected every month from approximately 27,000 outlets around the U.S.[17]

Items for which the prices are considered volatile—like groceries and electricity—are collected more often than others. For example, Figure 5.6A shows the price indices for the food and energy categories.[18] Both were considered volatile in the 1970s.

During President Richard Nixon's administration, there were complaints that the more fickle components of the CPI overshadowed the underlying price movements. That is, the inflation measure was wrong and inflation was actually lower. (This is very hard to determine!) And so, a version of the CPI-U was created with those bits removed. This index—CPI-U without food and energy—could be used to compute "core inflation."

12-month inflation for both versions of the CPI-U are graphed in Figure 5.6B. The two lines are hard to distinguish in the 1970s. Nevertheless, a few times, core inflation calculated in some manner was a bit lower than regular inflation. To make things sound better,

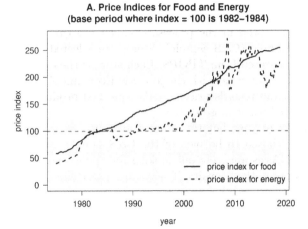

A. Price Indices for Food and Energy
(base period where index = 100 is 1982–1984)

B. 12–month Inflation Two Ways

Figure 5.6 Plot A shows the price indices for food and energy. As they are considered volatile components of the price index, a version of the CPI-U is published without them. Inflation calculated from that index is called "core inflation." Plot B shows two versions of inflation: CPI-U and with CPI-U without food and energy. Both are obtained by calculating the percent change between the index in a given month and the index in the same month in the previous year; both have also been seasonally adjusted. (Source: Bureau of Labor Statistics.)

the lower number was misleadingly given higher billing in government announcements.[88, 124] For us, the key feature the graph shows is that by removing two erratic components, food and energy, we are left with a (surprise!) less volatile price index.

(Given its charge to manage inflation, the Federal Reserve Bank previously tracked core inflation. In 2000, it decided to switch to using the Personal Consumption Expenditures Price Index calculated by the Bureau of Economic Analysis. It, too, has a "core" version.)

There are many exceptions to the basic C&S sample procedure, from postage to airline fares. For instance, people bargain when buying cars. Therefore, recording the sticker price would make cars seem costlier.

Computers are another example. The capabilities of PCs improve rapidly. Just like with apparel, items become obsolete frequently. PCs differ from clothing, however, because the capabilities of a computer change quickly too. And so, computers are handled in their own quirky way in the CPI.

Shelter—people's physical residence—is also priced separately. Initially, only rents were recorded. In 1953, BLS switched to using "homeowner costs" which included expenses from the price of the house to maintenance and repair costs.

The Stigler Commission (the same commission that suggesting moving away from the fixed basket formula), suggested that shelter be thought of as a "flow of services" rather than a good. The service they provide is, well, shelter. This idea was finally implemented in 1983 with a concept called "owner occupied rent" after many agencies (including BLS) and researchers endorsed it combined with more prosaic concerns about ballooning Social Security payments.[129]

Now, purchases of homes are not included in the CPI. Instead, shelter is priced using both rents for tenants and owner occupied rent for home owners. The latter is what a home owner would have been paying for rent had they been renting instead of owning. The CPI Housing Survey by BLS is used to obtain rental information and it, combined with data from the CE Survey, is used to calculate owner occupied rent.[17] (This is not the same as the American Housing Survey from the housing chapter.)

Collecting prices is complicated, varied, and time-intensive. There are adjustments to account for differences in quality, use of coupons, new products, and seasonality. These procedures were added and refined over time to improve inflation measurement.

CPI ≠ COST OF LIVING

While the idea of a price index has existed since the 1600s, cost of living indices are a far more recent invention. They are based on the bane of every Econ 101 student: utility functions. In essence, cost of living indices try to measure the cost of maintaining the same level of satisfaction (or utility) you derived from your purchases in the base period.

Utility functions are a theoretical idea and, in any case, differ from person to person because they reflect individual preferences. Therefore, a true cost of living index is impossible to calculate in real life regardless of how much effort you spend in curating a market basket of goods.

Price index formulas, however, can approximate them. For example, we know that people make substitutions in their spending when prices rise. Under those conditions, Laspeyres indices tend to overestimate the cost of living, whereas Paasche does the opposite. This makes Fisher's ideal price index, which is the geometric mean of the two, a better choice.[85]

Initially, the price index was called a cost of living index even though it really wasn't one at all. The CPI-U (or the CPI-W for that matter) was not designed to measure the true cost of living. That said, because of the 1961 Stigler Commission report, the goal of the CPI-U has slowly shifted to trying to approximate a cost of living index. This is what eventually precipitated the switch from the Laspeyres method to the EWGM method for calculating the CPI. The latter is considered a better approximation of cost of living.

In 2002, BLS began to publish a new type of price index, the Chained CPI-U (abbreviated as C-CPI-U) which better resembles a cost of living index. It makes use of the Törnqvist index, invented by the Finnish statistician Leo Törnqvist.

The key difference between the EWGM and Törnqvist methods is how the weights are calculated. An EWGM index uses weights based on older CE Survey data. On the other hand, the Törnqvist index requires current CE Survey data. That is, expenditure data collected concurrently with prices.

Given the lag between collecting data and publishing estimates, C-CPI-U values are more heavily revised as updated data becomes available. Consequently, it remains a supplemental measure, not the official one.

SUMMARY

Inflation is an important, lagging economic indicator in the U.S. It is calculated by computing the percent change in the CPI-U relative to its historical values. The CPI-U and CPI-W, the two consumer price indices, are produced by the Bureau of Labor Statistics using a wide number of data sources from the Consumer Expenditure Survey to the Commodities and Services sample. It has a variety of uses beyond tracking inflation, including determining Social Security payments. Given that processing survey data is time-intensive, there is a lag between data collection and publication. For example, the January 2019 price index values were published two weeks after the end of the month.

The CPI-U uses primarily an expenditure-share-weighted geometric mean (EWGM) formula, with a few items from the market basket indexed using the Laspeyres method. Basic product indices are computed, which are then combined to create the final, published indices.

The CPI-U is not a cost of living index although the goal is to approximate one. The market basket—the goods and services which are used in its calculations—is generated using aggregate expenditure information and not what a typical family would spend. It also represents only urban—not rural—consumers.

This gap between a household budget and aggregate amount spent can be problematic. The official numbers could indicate a low level of inflation, but people could be feeling that things are much worse when peering into their pocketbooks.

The procedures for determining the market basket, weights, and prices are extremely complex. This is because of the variety of similar product types, changes in spending habits, the addition of new product categories, and changes in product quality all have to be somehow incorporated. As a result, the definition of the CPI-U (and CPI-W) is continually in flux. However, these shifts are inevitable. Society keeps changing and so inflation measures must as well.

Janet Norwood, BLS Commissioner, said while testifying in front of Congress in the early 1980s, "Some people would like an index that doesn't go up so much, and other people would like an index that goes up more. And when they don't have that which they want, they feel there must be something wrong with the indicator itself."[78] This statement sums up much of inflation measurement history. Many changes were eventually implemented in response to political pressures, even though discussions about those changes had been tumbling about for many years.

FURTHER READING

The Cost of Living in America: A Political History of Economic Statistics, 1880–2000 by Thomas A. Stapleford. Cambridge University Press, 2009.

States, especially Massachusetts, were the first to produce labor statistics in the U.S. Eventually a federal department was created but it took time for economic information to be collected with any regularity and uniformity. Stapleford explains in this detailed history how economic crises highlighted the need for continual data collection.

"A history of technology, via the Consumer Price Index" by Adrienne LaFrance. *The Atlantic*, April 5, 2016.

From TVs to cinema to the internet, this article talks about how new technology slowly appears in CPI calculations reflecting the changing role of technology in American society.

The Billion Prices Project developed by the Massachusetts Institute of Technology's Sloane School of Management and Harvard Business School.

As seen in this chapter, producing the CPI is extraordinarily time- and labor-intensive. The researchers involved in this project are experimenting with ways of producing inflation measures using online prices. Computer programs can quickly and cheaply extract prices from retailers' websites, allowing for even daily price indices to be calculated. Such a procedure could become part of the BLS methodology in the future, especially if online and store pricing is similar.

CHAPTER 6

Poverty

4 OUNCES OF SALT PORK, 2 OUNCES OF BUTTER, 16 OUNCES OF BEANS, AND 8 OUNCES OF BREAD. This is a suggested daily intake for a "man at moderate muscular work." In 1894, this would have cost you less than 14 cents but provided a whopping 3,500 calories.[8]

This (scrumptious?) menu was suggested by W. O. Atwater as part of a U.S. Department of Agriculture report, marking the dawn of the food guide age.

Curiously, poverty measurement in the U.S. is based entirely on food costs, despite the (obvious) fact that food is not the only thing we need to survive. The cost of food is used to set an income threshold. If a family earns below this amount, everyone in that family is considered poor. The official poverty rate, then, is the percentage of population classified as poor.

This income threshold is also used to distribute federal funds to local governments and to determine a person's eligibility for programs such as Head Start and the Supplemental Nutrition Assistance Program (SNAP).

The debate on the causes of poverty across the centuries drifts continually among divine intervention, luck, systemic issues in society, and an individual's choices. These discussions influence how poverty is measured.

The principal divide in people's thinking is between absolute and relative poverty measures. An absolute measure just designates everyone who makes less than some amount (a threshold) as poor. The quickest example is the World Bank's memorable $1-a-day poverty line. (This line was later incorporated into the United Nations' global poverty reduction goals.)

It's easy to see why it's popular. One dollar is simple to remember. Moreover, life is extremely tough if that's all you have to live on. So it helps to evoke sad and pitiful imagery too.

This threshold—now $1.90-a-day having been adjusted for inflation—isn't concerned with whether that money can afford you a decent life or even enough food to eat. It was simply the number originally obtained by averaging poverty thresholds across fifteen countries deemed to be extremely poor.

The $1.90-a-day standard isn't versatile. For example, if that threshold was applied to, say, the U.S., it would appear as if there was virtually no poverty all. However, this is patently not true. A trek in any major U.S. city brings you into contact with the homeless.

This brings us to relative measures. These look a bit more like inequality measures. They focus on determining how well a person is doing in comparison to those around them.

The World Bank later turned their absolute threshold into a rudimentary relative one. Instead of using a single threshold, they use three: the original $1.90-a-day, $3.20-a-day, and $5.50-a-day. Each line applies to a different group of countries, depending on its income levels.[160] This is what makes the measure slightly more relative.

The $5.50-a-day line would apply to the U.S. If we multiply it by 365 days, we get an annual threshold of $2,008. This is a pretty low number. We can compare it to $12,488 per year, the 2017 official U.S. poverty threshold for an adult. It is considerably higher than $2,008.[34] So, while the $5.50 line is more relevant than $1.90, it's still very much on the low end.

Both absolute and relative measures are needed and useful. Nobel Laureate Amartya Sen reasoned that a relative measure is unhelpful if no one has enough to eat and an absolute one isn't useful if everyone does. However, if you use the absolute measure for ensuring physical needs are met and a relative one to see how well someone can participate in the society they live in, a clearer picture of society can emerge.[138] (Keep this idea in mind as you read this chapter.)

The curious nature of the U.S. poverty measure requires some historical context because, as mentioned earlier, it is entirely dependent on food costs. This is the focus of the next section, but the timeline in Figure 6.1 provides a quick summary.

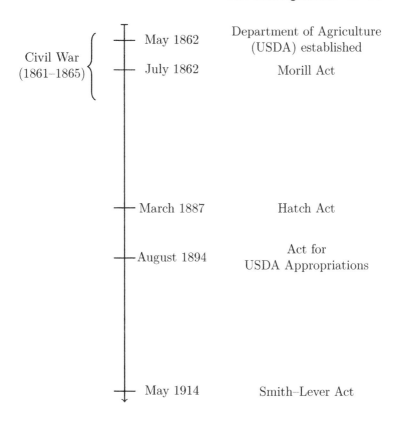

Figure 6.1 Congressional acts which set the scene for developing a poverty measure based on food costs.

ALL ABOUT AGRICULTURE

Amidst the cannon fire and smoke of the Civil War, President Abraham Lincoln created the U.S. Department of Agriculture (USDA). A few months later, he signed the Morill Act.

The Morill Act offered federal land to states to sell. States could then use those proceeds to establish a land-grant college. (Iowa State University was the first such college.) This superb opportunity was open only to Northern states, since, conveniently, they hadn't seceded. Part of this was likely an attempt by Lincoln to widen the divide between Northern and Southern states, culminating in the Emancipation Proclamation which freed the slaves.

These efforts produced a burst of scientific activity. This only increased when agriculture experimental stations were set up at land-grant colleges in 1887 when the Hatch Act was passed. The aim was to encourage research about farming from animal diseases to experiments on fertilizer types.

The connection to land-grant colleges was twofold. First, these colleges had a natural source of expertise through their faculty. Second, having facilities scattered across the country would allow research agendas to reflect the needs of local farming environments.[53]

(These laws show that the federal government was enthusiastic about promoting *farming*. This enthusiasm, it must be noted, did not necessarily extend to *farmers*. Various developments and governmental policies made life difficult for the average farmer, many of whom ended up becoming tenants on their own farms. Eventually, they formed unions, contributing to the burgeoning populist movement in the late 1800s.[165])

Soon this research led to studies on nutrition, linking diet to health. Here is where Atwater enters the story.

Wilbur Olin Atwater was a chemistry professor at Wesleyan University in Connecticut, a pioneer in nutrition studies and—for better or for worse—calorie counting.

In August 1894, Congress passed an appropriations act for the USDA. Most of this was ho hum, routine government stuff: $1,200 for hiring a telegraph and telephone operator, $3,000 to study soil samples. (Incidentally, the act also made it illegal to publish false weather reports especially if you said they came from the Weather Bureau.)

In the middle of all of this, $10,000 was set aside to produce a report on nutrition, food waste, and food costs.[50] Atwater was hired to write the report. In it, he incorporated costs to assemble what, at the time, would have been considered healthy menus.[8]

Research activities burbled along until May 1914 when President Woodrow Wilson signed the Smith–Lever Act.[53] Now, the USDA added the dissemination of its research to the general public to its mission. One effect of the act was to establish the Cooperative Extension Service which provided vocational training. Another effect—the bit relevant to us—was bringing nutrition information to the average American.

During World War I, Caroline Hunt, a nutritionist at USDA, published the department's first nutrition guide for children and another shortly after for adults.[84] Some of the advice should sound familiar: Drink milk! Finish your vegetables! Chew slowly!

These guides were updated periodically, offering families fresh information about how to eat healthily. (Food pyramids and My-Plate are the modern versions of these guides.)

A few decades later, the Great Depression hit. Staggering levels of unemployment meant many people went hungry. As we know, this was around the time President Franklin D. Roosevelt started to mandate consistent collection of unemployment data.

He also commissioned the 1935–1936 Study of Consumer Purchases to examine nearly every angle of family expenses. A concerted attempt was made to choose families who were representative of different types of living—rural, farming, urban, etc. On the other hand, there was a clear emphasis on surveying primarily white families where both the husband and wife were born in the country in the dubious interests of "homogeneity." (To give some context, according to the 1930 census, 11.6% of the population was foreign born and around 10.6% of people were born in the U.S. but not white.[36])

Researchers poured over data on income earned and spending on housing, clothing, transportation, medical care, and so forth. Additionally, they calculated food expenses by income level, family size, and race. It was found that less than one-third of American families were eating (and could afford) what was deemed a "good" diet. The remaining two-thirds of families had either "fair" or "poor" diets.[146] This was not a cheery result.

Soon World War II began and even though the U.S. officially entered after the attack on Pearl Harbor, preparations had already commenced quietly. Based on the 1935–1936 Study of Consumer Purchases, Roosevelt organized the National Nutrition Conference for Defense at the end of May in 1941. (Pearl Harbor was bombed in December.) While the event was being planned, he stated, "Total defense demands manpower. The full energy of every American is necessary...every man and woman in America must have nourishing food."[110] (This conference, incidentally, was also where recommended daily allowances (RDAs) of nutrients originated.)

Making sure people were properly fed had become a national security issue. And so, more resources were devoted to studying nutrition and giving advice on suitable menus especially in response to food rations during the war. Figure 6.2 on page 102 is a good example of a patriotic appeal to Americans.[155]

While establishing the USDA was the first step in the long march to promoting nutritious diets, this was doubly reinforced during World War II by the maxim, hungry people = weak nation.

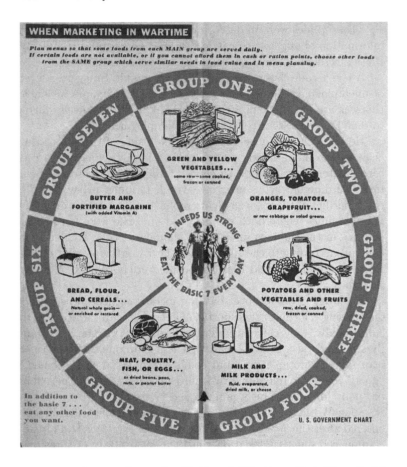

Figure 6.2 A page from the *National Wartime Nutrition Guide* published in July 1943. (Source: U.S. Department of Agriculture.)

In practical terms, this meant that there was a lot of information about food and its costs drifting around the corridors of government. This was information which could be used to develop a poverty measure.

FOOD × 3

Mollie Orshansky, who worked at the Social Security Administration, started to develop a poverty measure in 1963 as part of her research. Her statistic was designed to make use of the best available data at that time: nutrients required for a balanced diet along with food expenditures.

The 1960s were a time of great social change in the U.S.: The Civil Rights movement, protests against the Vietnam War, the women's liberation movement, immigration reform, the Cold War, the space race.

It was also the decade of President Lyndon B. Johnson's "unconditional war on poverty." Johnson made this declaration during his first State of the Union address in January of 1964, asserting that, "The richest Nation on earth can afford to win it. We cannot afford to lose it." In his speech, Johnson listed plans from expanding the food stamp program to creating what became Medicare (health insurance for the elderly), from overhauling taxes to spur job creation to establishing relief projects in the Appalachian Mountains.[87] (Unfortunately, this figurative war came to a swift end due to the rising costs of a literal one, the Vietnam War.[113])

As with unemployment, if anything was to be done about poverty, some form of measurement was needed to decide who was poor, who qualified for social programs, and whether things were getting better or worse. After Johnson's speech, the Office of Economic Opportunity ferreted about, found Orshansky's work, and adopted it as the official measure.

Poverty measures have two components. First, there must be a way to establish an income threshold, a monetary amount below which people are counted as poor. Second, that threshold must then be applied to income data to determine the poverty rate.

Orshansky dealt with the first issue by combining the following using results from the 1955 Food Consumption Survey:

- Approximately 1/3 of a household's after-tax income was spent on food.[94]

- The Economy Food Plan, designed by the USDA, provided necessary nutrients cheaply.[49]

(Unlike the 1935–1936 Study of Consumer Purchases, the 6,000 households interviewed in 1955 were intended to represent everyone in the country, apart from Alaska and Hawaii which were yet to become states.[55])

And so, the national poverty threshold for a household is:[120]

$$\text{today's poverty threshold} = \left(\text{cost of Economy Food Plan in 1963} \times 3 \right) \times \text{today's inflation adjustment}.$$

Multiplying the cost of the Economy Food Plan by three is a rough estimate of a household's after-tax income. That number is then updated annually to account for inflation using the CPI-U to get the current poverty threshold.

(Remember, U stands for the urban consumer. Today, over 80% of the U.S. population is considered to be living in an urban environment. At the time of writing, President Donald J. Trump's administration was toying with the idea of replacing CPI-U with another inflation measure, such as CPI-W, C-CPI-U, or the price index produced by the Bureau of Economic Analysis.[116])

Finally, residents of households with incomes which are below that threshold are classified as poor. The percentage of people classified as poor is the poverty rate.

1963 is the key year for the official poverty rate. This is the same year the Beatles released their first album, Valentina Tershkova from the USSR became the first woman to go to space, and Martin Luther King Jr. gave his "I have a dream" speech at the March on Washington. This is also the year AT&T Bell System introduced touch-tone dialing on landline telephones, President John F. Kennedy was assassinated, and Kenya became an independent country.[118] A humble formula for a monumental year.

Orshansky's formula is applied to pre-tax income, even though the original 1/3 statistic was calculated after taxes were deducted. She opined that at the low end of the income distribution, this simplification would not make much of a difference.

In 2017, the official threshold was $24,858 for a family of four, including two related children.[42] It was then modified, based on the size of the family, when calculating the poverty rate. Initially, the threshold was also lowered for farming families, the rationale being that people who grew some of their own food spent less on food. This farm adjustment, however, was eventually dropped.

Today, household income data from the Annual Social and Economic Supplement to the Current Population Survey (CPS) is used to calculate the percentage of people in poverty. The CPS is administered monthly by the Census Bureau—this is also where the unemployment numbers come from—but the supplement is tacked on only a few times throughout the year.

We can see how this percentage has changed each year in Figure 6.3. The poverty rate was over 20% at the start of the 1960s, steadily decreasing across the decade. Since then, according to this measure, the rate has never reached as high, although it has fluctuated over time.[34]

U.S. Poverty Rates

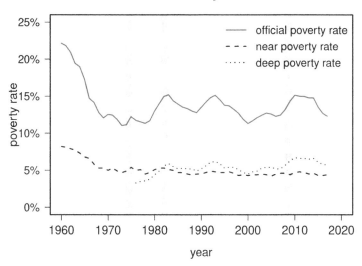

Figure 6.3 Annual U.S. poverty rate (solid) which gives the percentage of people "in poverty" (the official poverty rate); the percentage of people "near poverty" (dash), who earn between between 100% and 125% of the poverty threshold; and the percentage of people in "deep poverty" (dot), who earn less than 50% of the poverty threshold. Even though the measure was developed with 1963 as the base year, it was applied back to 1959. The shaded areas represent the major recessions in the U.S.: after the 1973 and 1979 oil crises and the Great Recession which began in December 2007. (Sources: Annual Social and Economic Supplement to the Current Population Survey; National Bureau of Economic Research.)

CPS is designed to provide data sufficient for producing good national estimates. Within any given county, for example, only a few households, if any, are contacted to participate in the survey. And so, CPS isn't practical for calculating poverty rates for smaller regions like counties or school districts. For that, the Census Bureau applies the national poverty threshold to data from the American Community Survey (ACS) to obtain local poverty rates using statistical models. This procedure is called the Small Area Income and Poverty Estimates (SAIPE) program. Results from SAIPE are used to allocate federal funding locally.

Let's go back to Figure 6.3. The official poverty rate was given by the solid line. But there are two other lines on this graph. The dashed line shows the percentage of people whose family income is between the threshold and 25% above the threshold. These are people whose family income makes them "near poverty." The dotted line tracks people considered to be in "deep poverty," who are a subset of those counted as poor. These people live in households with a family income less than 50% of the threshold.

The near and deep poverty classifications are calculated by taking a family's income and dividing it by the threshold. This give us the "ratio of income to poverty." At the family level, this ratio can be used as a criterion for determining whether a particular family qualifies for governmental benefits. We will discuss one example here: food stamps.

In 1928, Henry A. Wallace, editor in chief of the newspaper *Wallaces' Farmer*, went on the radio to note the irony that the USDA and the experimental stations at land-grant universities spent a lot of effort improving agricultural productivity, only to have it result in surplus goods making it difficult for farmers to sell their harvests. He said, "If this continues another 10 years, I would not be surprised. . .to see many farmers rise up in their anger and demand that the government spend its money on making city people efficient rather than farmers."[142]

He was right. By 1933, farmers were producing too much and were unable to recoup their expenses as the surpluses meant that prices dropped. Simultaneously, thanks to the effects of the Great Depression, many families were hungry.

Wallace, by this time Secretary of Agriculture (he later became Roosevelt's Vice President), had several solutions. He started with the 1933 Agricultural Adjustment Act which paid farmers to reduce how much they planted, especially cotton, wheat, and corn. Livestock and crops were also destroyed to reduce the total supply.

Another solution was food stamps, a way for Roosevelt to kill two birds with one stone. The edible surplus would be given to the poor. This scheme was formalized in 1939 and called the Food Stamp Program.

First deployed in Rochester, New York, the program proceeded as follows: People paid $1 for an orange stamp that could be used like cash to buy food. Along with that orange stamp, they would get a free 50 cent blue stamp that could be used only to buy goods on the surplus list.

What the blue stamps could buy kept changing based on what was considered a surplus good. In May of 1939, you could get things like butter, oranges, and corn meal. Oranges were removed from the list in July of that year when onions were added, but were back on the list by December.

The whole thing was quite complicated, but was designed so that people spent their usual amount on food (the orange stamps) and then supplemented that amount with extra food (the blue stamps). The program was eventually halted when the war effort kick-started the economy and the surplus problem vanished.[121]

Food stamps resurfaced and eventually became a formal program in 1964 when President Johnson signed the Food Stamp Act as part of his war on poverty. The program has changed since then, and in 2008 was renamed the Supplemental Nutrition Assistance Program (SNAP). This name change was in part because stamps were dropped and replaced with an Electronic Benefits Transfer (EBT) Card, which acts like a debit card. Orshansky's poverty threshold, however, is still used to determine whether you are eligible for SNAP.[29]

So we see the poverty threshold is used at three levels: to calculate a national poverty rate, to allocate federal funding at the local level by applying the threshold to more granular data, and to determine eligibility for governmental programs.

A FORK IN THE ROAD

Throughout the evolution of the U.S. poverty measure, it has remained an absolute measure. Europe went another way, even though at the start, there were some similar ideas. In the late 1800s, however, ideas floated between Britain and the U.S. with regards to the study of poverty.

For example, Charles Booth conducted a comprehensive study of life in London, publishing numerous volumes on topics from unemployment to religion.

He also produced a striking map of London poverty levels. Each road, street, terrace, crescent, mews, and so on was painstakingly color-coded. Residents whose homes bordered Hyde Park were wealthy. Families living on Eastbourne Terrace by Paddington

Railway Station were considered merely well-to-do. The opposite side of the station housed poorer residents.

Booth's classifications were based on things like whether a family had servants or if their earnings were regular or intermittent. In addition to income, he also studied expenditures on food (tea included, of course), housing, clothing, and "fire and light," among other things.

That said, to modern eyes, despite its thoroughness and stacks of tables, Booth's calculations were fuzzy and unscientific, relying heavily on ethnographic-type field work and on the "expert opinions" of local school board members. For example, his categorization of Londoners ranged from the posh "Upper middle and Upper classes. Wealthy." to the riffraff, described as "Lowest class. Vicious, semi-criminal."[96]

Booth's work was an inspiration for the similarly-detailed Hull House Maps and Papers depicting a Chicago settlement house. Chicago's maps, however, focused more on wages and race rather than poverty directly. They were commissioned by the Bureau of Labor Statistics (BLS) as part of a larger study and were overseen by local labor activist Florence E. Kelley, who actually lived in Hull House.[113]

In the reverse direction, Benjamin Seebohm Rowntree, in his study of poverty in York, England, used our calorie-counter friend Atwater's work. Specifically, in his 1901 publication, Rowntree reconfigured Atwater's caloric recommendations to formulate what looked a lot like the Economy Food Plan used in Orshansky's measure.

In addition to food, he looked at costs for rent, clothing, light and fuel, trying to ascertain the minimum expenditures necessary for survival. He also made allowances for "household sundries" (soap, utensils). In subsequent studies he added the "personal sundries" category which included a rather wide range of items from National Health Insurance, newspapers, and stamps, along with beer, tobacco, and, "occasional presents to the children."[134]

Rowntree applied his minimum expenditure budget to incomes from families he surveyed to create two categories: primary and secondary poverty. Those in primary poverty did not earn enough to afford the items included in Rowntree's minimum budget; those in secondary poverty could, but failed to plan appropriately. His decision about whom to put where was relatively unscientific, relying on personal observation and help from (possibly nosy) neighbors.[133]

Despite the initial cross-pollination of ideas, it appears that subsequently there was little interaction between camps. The U.S. went along its route to Orshansky's poverty measure, an absolute measure which only looked at the cost of food. Meanwhile in Europe, developments in poverty research veered to relative measures. The American Dream, the belief that one lives in a meritocratic society with an expectation of pulling yourself up by your bootstraps, lends itself naturally to an absolute poverty measure. Such measures set the bar at basic survival, as climbing above that point would be up to your own efforts.[12]

Thinking about costs for food, shelter, and so forth make sense if there is a significant proportion of the population who has trouble affording a subsistence-level life. (Like the World Bank's $1.90-a-day threshold.) To participate in society requires being able to afford those items. For richer countries, however, participation in society goes beyond physical necessities and could include education, access to internet, and indoor plumbing.

To recall Amartya Sen's argument from the start of this chapter, the absolute threshold may be most useful for clearing the low bar of being able to stay alive. He suggests a relative approach after that to take into account standards of living within a society. The European outlook follows this vein of thought.

The organization tasked with putting together a poverty measure for the European Economic Community announced a "War on Want" in 1975, evoking Johnson's similar pronouncement a decade earlier: "...individuals and families are described as beset by poverty when their 'resources are so small as to exclude them from the minimum acceptable way of life of the Member State in which they live.' "[68]

This definition does not stop at basic subsistence; it explicitly takes into account standards of living. Sen pointed out that this is not a new idea, noting even economist Adam Smith (with his infamous invisible hand) considered standards of living in his book, *The Wealth of Nations*.[138]

Since 1975, the countries within the European Union have focused on developing many types of relative poverty measures, published through the agency Eurostat. For instance, they define their "risk-of-poverty threshold" to be 60% of the median income of a country (welfare benefits included).[69] (Remember that the median is the income at which half of the population earns more, and the other half earns less.) This is a relative measure because we aren't looking at what are considered minimum costs, but rather the bottom segment of society.

Another type of relative calculation is a deprivation measure. These take a holistic approach to poverty and participation in society by looking at factors such as whether people own their home. We will discuss them in the next chapter.

A potential downside of relative measures—for countries where subsistence living is uncommon—is it is difficult to ascertain whether poverty has increased or decreased over time. This is because as incomes rise, the threshold also rises. However, given that the goals of European Union poverty measures consider standards of living, this is less of an immediate issue, and simply requires one to do a bit more analysis with the data.

CHECKLISTS

When developing her absolute poverty measure, Orshansky had to satisfy the following list of requirements:

1. Define what it means to be a "family."

2. Determine how to calculate the poverty threshold.

3. Specify how to adjust that threshold depending at the very least on family size.

4. Decide what counts as income.

5. Choose how often the measure should be computed (e.g., every month, year) and at which geographic level (e.g., national, state).[12]

To improve the U.S. poverty measure, we would need better answers to the items in this checklist.

Items 1, 3, and 5 are mostly technical points. Technical points, however, can have big impacts.

For example, a family could be defined as related people who live together in houses or apartments. This seems reasonable. It also matches up with the colloquial definition of the word "family." However, this strict definition actually leaves people out such as foster kids living with people they aren't related to. People in jail or in college dorms don't fit in either.

Like the unemployment rate, the poverty rate is the ratio of people in poverty divided by all people. Those not counted in the family definition are left out of both the top and bottom values, possibly distorting the results.

Defining income (point 4 in the checklist) isn't clear-cut, either. Currently, income is measured pre-tax, even though Orshansky's original formula was based on post-tax income.

Income from capital gains isn't included. Neither is non-cash government assistance, like housing subsidies. Many of these government programs nudge families *out of poverty*. The results of those efforts don't show up in the measure.

In practice, both types of information would be helpful: The first to see the state of things, the second to see how much welfare programs have achieved in reducing poverty.

These examples are minor compared to the elephant in the room: defining the poverty threshold (point 2). The purpose of the threshold is to determine how much money is needed to survive. Somehow, a family needs to cobble together that much after-tax income. (This is separate from point 4, which is how to add up people's earnings to compare them to the threshold.)

We could think about what people *ought* to be spending versus what people actually spend their money on. However, reasonable people could have widely differing views on this front.

In the official poverty measure, both perspectives were used. First, Orshansky used the observation that approximately one-third of after-tax income was used on food. This considers what people are actually doing with their money, at least what they were doing in the 1950s.

Then, she used the cost of the Economy Food Plan to construct her threshold. Implicit in this (well-intentioned) proposition is that this is what low-income households ought to be eating and paying for their food. However, the procedure ignores whether that is possible in the current year or a given city.

Geographic adjustments for the poverty threshold, beyond urban and rural, which anyway were eventually dropped, were deemed too difficult due to a lack of reliable information consistently available for the entire country.

Given all of these flaws, we are probably all wondering why this measure still exists in its fossilized 1963 form. Even Orshansky was disconcerted it was the official statistic, writing that, "The best you can say for the measure is that at a time when it seemed useful, it was there."[119]

We can thank the Office of Management and Budget (OMB), part of the executive branch of the federal government, for this decision. In 1969, the government required poverty calculations to be published and Orshansky's measure was adopted. Then, in 1978, the OMB's Statistical Policy Directive No. 14 forced the Census Bureau to stick with her formula.[12, 115]

To change this policy, requires a lot of effort on the part of the executive branch. Small changes in the threshold could result in radically different numbers of people in poverty. Moreover, programs like SNAP, which we talked about earlier, depend on this official measure. Changing the measure would then affect funding allocations as well. It's easy to see why this is a politically thorny issue and that there is little incentive to mess with the formula.[12] However, at the time of writing, the Trump administration was soliciting comments about changing the inflation measure used in poverty rate calculations (see page 104).

However—and this is the silver lining here—Directive No. 14 did allow for people to experiment with other measures, even though they couldn't be used to distribute federal funds or anything else official.

This left the door wide open for new ideas. An updated poverty threshold would need fresh answers to three questions:

• What items are required to live a decent life?

• What is the reasonable, minimum cost for these items each year?

• Should the calculations be made differently depending on where in the country you live?

To get a sense of what choices seem sensible, let's look at some BLS data about how people spend their money from the 2016–2017 Consumer Expenditure Survey.[20]

As mentioned in the chapter on prices and inflation, this survey uses "consumer units," which is a more general version of "family." For our purposes, it also means we don't have a direct match between the groupings of people when measuring poverty officially and the groupings of people in this data. We can still get a general lay of the land with this information, however.

To start, let's divide the U.S. into four regions: Northeast, Midwest, South, and West (see Figure 6.4). This split is not equitable by the number of states, number of residents, or even land mass. It's just the distribution set by the Census Bureau for reporting purposes and roughly matches colloquial notions of areas of the country. The data we will look at will be parsed by region.

Regions in the U.S.

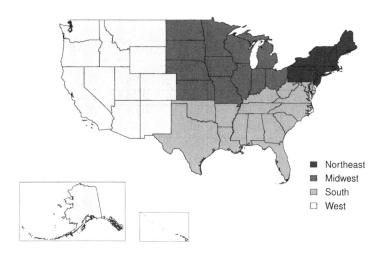

Figure 6.4 This map shows the four "regions" of the U.S. as designated by the Census Bureau. While Washington, D.C. is included as part of the "South," Puerto Rico and the other U.S. territories are excluded. (Alaska and Hawaii are not to scale in this map.) (Source: Census Bureau, Geography Division.)

We know that people at different life stages have different needs. For example, children need to go to school, see the pediatrician, and have someone take care of them. They may eventually attend college, move out of the house, and get married. We also know that the cost of living differs across the U.S. and jobs are not distributed evenly.

For now, let's focus on the segment of the population which earns between $50,000 and $69,999 per year. (Here, income includes things like pensions and government benefits.) Before we look at expenditures, we should first get an idea about what types of people have incomes in this range.

Table 6.5 provides some information about the consumer units in each region. For example, the South has the most number of

TABLE 6.5 This table summarizes the composition of consumer units in each region who earn between $50,000 and $69,999 before paying taxes. Consumer units are an expanded version of a family; they include unrelated individuals (i.e., the "consumers") who make most of their financial decisions jointly (i.e., "the unit"). (Source: 2016–2017 Consumer Expenditure Survey.)

	Northeast	Midwest	South	West
no. of consumer units (in millions)	2.91	3.75	6.42	3.88
avg. unit size	2.40	2.54	2.64	2.74
avg. no. under 18	0.49	0.61	0.65	0.71
avg. no. 65 and older	0.40	0.35	0.32	0.37

units, but the average size of a unit is larger in the West. The Northeast has the lowest number of children per unit on average, but the highest average number of people qualifying for senior citizen discounts per unit.

Turning to Figure 6.6, we can see how these consumer units spend their money on average every year. Each bar graph depicts a type of expense and each bar corresponds to one of the four regions. These are not the top expenses for a consumer unit, just a mix of things that are necessary, like housing, or fun, like reading.

Midwesterners, perhaps stereotypically, spend the most on dairy products. Northeasterners appear to have the most expensive housing, but Westerners are a close second. The latter also seem to spend more on both reading materials and their pets. Southerners spend the least on alcohol.

The consumer units represented in this graph earn approximately the same amount of money, but appear to live very different lifestyles, a mixture of choice and necessity.

Some choices are practical: you must have heating to survive Maine winters. Others are lifestyle-based: vegans manage without eggs.

Despite these individual choices, the cost of living differs across the U.S. Therefore, you cannot simply plant your $100,000 New York City salary into Chicago and plan to upgrade from a studio apartment to a house with a yard. You may have to take a pay cut to live in Omaha, settling for a two-bedroom apartment, perhaps. How much you are better off can be a tricky calculation.

The Census Bureau calculates local poverty rates through the SAIPE program. The catch is that the national poverty threshold

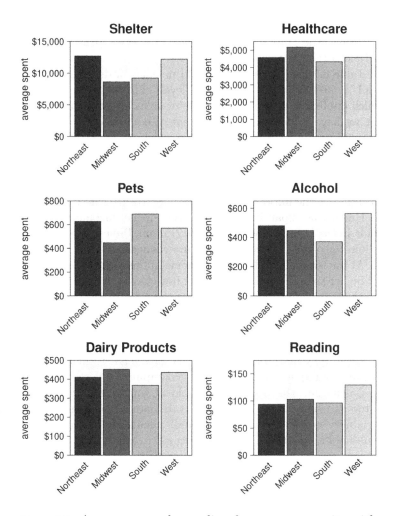

Figure 6.6 Average annual spending for consumer units with a pre-tax income, which includes pensions and government benefits, between $50,000 and $69,999 each year. Regional differences across the U.S. are noticeable for various types of expenditures, from where to live to what to eat. Note that the vertical axis scale is different across plots. (Source: 2016–2017 Consumer Expenditure Survey.)

is still applied. This means, if the threshold is $25,000, it is applied to incomes the same way in San Francisco (very expensive) as it is in Helena (far cheaper). Table 6.7 lists median household incomes in different parts of the U.S. and at various geographic levels. This data is from ACS, which publishes income information for areas like states and cities, but we have to deal with the concept of households. For poverty estimates, we focused on the family, which requires people to be related; then, we used the consumer unit for the expenditure data which includes unrelated individuals, provided they made a lot of their financial decisions together. Now, we have the household, the most general definition of all: people who live together.

Under this expansive definition, the median income for households in the U.S. was $60,336 in 2017. From Table 6.7, we can see at lower geographic levels, the picture changes.

At the regional level, median income in the Northeast and West are higher than the national median. If we look at states, Maryland has the highest median household income at $80,776, whereas West Virginia has the lowest at $43,469. Both are far from $60,336, the national median. At the city level, metropolitan and micropolitan areas (smaller cities and towns), incomes are even more variable.[45]

Geography matters, that much is clear. What is unclear is the granularity required to account for geographical differences.

Calculating the poverty threshold at only the national level is too coarse because it does not take into account geographic variability at all. On the other hand, calculating poverty at the household level—that is, determining on a case-by-case basis who is poor—while, accounting for the variability across living conditions, is obviously not a practical solution. We need something in the middle.

SUPPLEMENTAL STATISTICS

In the 1990s, Congress disbursed funds to study poverty measures. They couldn't change the official measure because of the rules (remember Statistical Policy Directive No. 14), but they were allowed to experiment and publish alternatives.[48] Enter the Supplemental Poverty Measure (SPM) in 2011, during President Barack Obama's administration.

The SPM is more intricate compared to the official measure to accommodate the fact that life is complicated and highly varied. However, it's less elaborate than what the original panel envisioned

TABLE 6.7 This table lists the median household income in 2017 at various geographic levels, starting at the national level. Urban areas are divided into Core Based Statistical Areas (CBSAs). These are then split into Metropolitan Statistical Areas which contain an urban cluster with more than 50,000 residents and Micropolitan Statistical Areas which have an urban cluster containing between 10,000 and 50,000 residents. (Source: 2017 American Community Survey 1-year estimates.)

Level	Geography	Median Income ($)
nation	U.S.	60,336
region	Northeast	66,998
	Midwest	57,778
	South	55,135
	West	66,485
state	Alaska (AK)	73,181
	California (CA)	71,805
	Maryland (MD)	80,776
	Massachusetts (MA)	77,385
	Mississippi (MS)	43,529
	North Dakota (ND)	61,843
	Ohio (OH)	54,021
	West Virginia (WV)	43,469
urban core	Anchorage, AK Metro	76,871
	Athens, OH Micro	44,247
	Baltimore-Columbia-Towson, MD Metro	77,394
	Bluefield, WV-VA Micro	35,964
	Boston-Cambridge-Newton, MA-NH Metro	85,691
	Columbus, OH Metro	63,764
	Eureka-Arcata-Fortuna, CA Micro	46,494
	Fargo, ND-MN Metro	63,353
	Grand Forks, ND-MN Metro	48,609
	Greenfield Town, MA Micro	58,824
	Jackson, MS Metro	52,434
	Laurel, MS Micro	38,542
	San Diego-Carlsbad, CA Metro	76,207
	San Jose-Sunnyvale-Santa Clara, CA Metro	117,474
	Washington-Arlington-Alexandria, DC-VA-MD-WV Metro	99,669
	Weirton-Steubenville, WV-OH Metro	45,971

because not all of the desired data was available. (Of course, this could change in the future and the SPM would probably be updated.)

The first step—as with Orshansky's measure and our checklists—is to define what counts as a family. The SPM uses a more inclusive definition of family than the official poverty rate does. For example, kids under 15 who aren't related to the adults in the house are excluded from the family unit; the SPM adds them back in.

Next up is defining the poverty threshold. The rationale here is to add up four things that people need to survive: food, clothing, shelter, and utilities (e.g., electricity, phone, water), then add a bit more for miscellaneous expenses (e.g., school supplies, towels, spatulas).

This list should sound familiar. If we replace "utilities" for "fuel and light," we have Rowntree's original expenditure list, with a buffer added which essentially accounts for his household and personal sundries component. (Booth also looked at a similar collection of items in his poverty studies.)

In any case, these four spending categories join to form the catchy acronym FCSU. Instead of tallying how much money people ought to be spending on food or housing, cues are taken from actual spending behavior.

FCSU expenditures across different income groups are graphed in Figure 6.8 for consumer units containing any combination of four people.[20] Each bar in this graph represents an income range from lowest to highest. The boxes within a bar represent average spending on one of the four items; the white box represents all other expenses.

It's not surprising that the "other expenditures" box balloons as incomes rise—people who earn more have more disposable income. They have more money to spend on holidays and the theater, private school, cars, and healthcare.

Food expenditures, in contrast, stay relatively steady until the highest income ranges, possibly reflecting eating out more or buying organic or specialty foods. Contrary to the consumption study results from the 1950s, food now comprises, on average, less than one-third of a household's expenses.

Housing and utilities expenses are reasonably stable as well until the highest income ranges. For utilities, a higher income means you could spend more money on better data plans or cool a larger

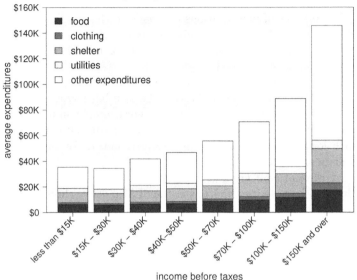

Figure 6.8 Average expenditures by income for a four-person consumer unit, which is not necessarily two adults and two kids. These expenditures are split into the FCSU categories—food, clothing, shelter, and utilities—and a miscellaneous expenses category. (Source: 2016–2017 Consumer Expenditure Survey.)

house. (Remember these are *average* expenditures which means that specific consumer units may be spending more or less.)

Building a minimum budget akin to the Economy Food Plan for these FCSU items requires a slew of assumptions. Instead, the SPM uses actual expenditures. To ensure a sufficient amount of data, five years worth of expenditure surveys are combined after adjusting for inflation. (This is exactly what we did in the housing chapter. To have an adequate number of home sales per time period, we created a quarterly index instead of a monthly one.)

From the merged data, the point which splits the bottom third from the top two-thirds (the 33rd percentile) is selected. This quantity is deemed to be the "reasonable" minimum amount to spend on FCSU. It is then multiplied by 1.2 to account for other expenses.

This is the baseline threshold and is updated annually with current expenditure data.[74]

Three types of modifications are made to this baseline threshold. First, it's adjusted for family size and composition. We know that a similar sort of adjustment is made for the official poverty measure, so no surprises there.

Second, families are assigned to one of three categories: those who rent, those who own, and those who own but pay a mortgage. Costs differ among these three settings. For example, in more rural areas people are more likely to own their home without a mortgage, which lowers their housing costs. Not accounting for that would result in an artificially high poverty rate.[48, 74]

At the national level, for a family of four with two children living in a house with a mortgage, the SPM poverty threshold was $27,085 in 2017.

This number is then fine-tuned depending on housing costs in defined areas corresponding to population hubs. To get a sense of these geographic adjustments, see Figure 6.9 which shows California and Ohio as examples.[128]

Each region represents either a metropolitan area, a micropolitan area, or neither (too small to count as either). The first two are called Core Based Statistical Areas (CBSA), which we first talked about in the housing chapter. These are not legal boundaries, just the Census Bureau's approximation of what people think of as commuter zones or population hubs. They can extend beyond city limits and even state borders.

For example, the New York City has five boroughs: Manhattan, the Bronx, Brooklyn, Queens, and Staten Island. However, the metropolitan area includes communities in Westchester County in the state, but not city, of New York, along with parts of New Jersey and Connecticut. This is why the state of Ohio in Figure 6.9 has extra bits which extend into Pennsylvania, West Virginia, Kentucky, and Indiana.

California is home to Silicon Valley, one of the most expensive places to live. It's the white blob southeast of San Francisco on the map and represents the area around San Jose. (To afford these expensive homes, you need a lot of money; we saw in Table 6.7 that the median income in San Jose is $117,474.)

In contrast, Ohio is far cheaper, which is why its SPM poverty thresholds are lower. The highest thresholds are for the three largest cities in the state: Columbus, Cleveland, and Cincinnati.

Supplemental Poverty Measure Thresholds in California

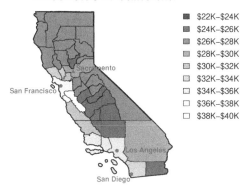

- ■ $22K–$24K
- ■ $24K–$26K
- ■ $26K–$28K
- ▨ $28K–$30K
- ▨ $30K–$32K
- ▢ $32K–$34K
- ▢ $34K–$36K
- ▢ $36K–$38K
- ▢ $38K–$40K

Supplemental Poverty Measure Thresholds in Ohio

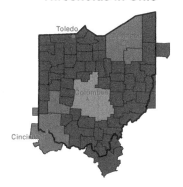

Figure 6.9 The 2017 national poverty threshold for the Supplemental Poverty Measure for families with two adults and two children living in a home they own, but with a mortgage, is $27,085. This threshold is then adjusted to account for regional housing costs. The resulting threshold ranges for areas in California and Ohio are mapped here. Major cities are marked along with the state capitals (triangles). (Sources: Bureau of Labor Statistics; Census Bureau, Geography Division.)

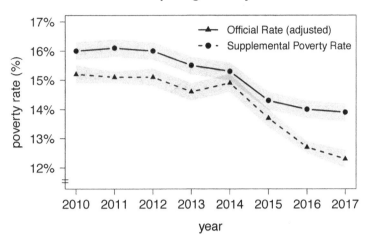

Figure 6.10 Estimates of the poverty rate from 2010 to 2017 using two definitions: the official rate (triangles with dotted lines) and the Supplemental Poverty Measure (circles with solid lines). The official rate has been adjusted so that the definition of a family is similar to that used in the supplemental one. Given the other differences in definitions, however, it is better to compare trends rather than the actual values. The bands around the plotted points represent 90% confidence intervals, providing information about the precision of the poverty rate estimates. (Source: Census Bureau.)

Figure 6.10 compares the official poverty measure with the SPM from 2010 to 2017. The official rate has been adjusted so that its definition of family is similar to the one used in the SPM.[73]

We need to be careful comparing these numbers because even though they both "measure poverty," the definitions of what it means to be poor, as we've seen, differ substantially. Instead, we should check whether or not the estimates are moving in the same direction. That is, we should compare trends: Over the last few years, both measures are slowly decreasing.

We've talked about Booth and Rowntree. The third man in this succession of British researchers is Sir Arthur Lyon Bowley.

He took the work of his predecessors and tried to make it more scientific by surveying a random sample of households to estimate economic statistics in the early 1900s. He was also the first to introduce the idea of using measures of precision in social science research; previously, it was mostly used in the natural sciences.[14]

Looking again to Figure 6.10, the shaded bands around each series represent information about the precision of the poverty estimates. These are what are called 90% confidence interval bands. For each year, we have a poverty estimate and along with that, we can compute a confidence interval. This is the measure of precision.

You've probably seen confidence intervals before in election poll results under the guise of plus or minus some amount of percentage points.

For example, if candidate Holmes is projected to win 52% of the vote against candidate Watson according to a poll, it looks like Holmes is going to win. This percentage is estimated using a small sample of likely voters, not by asking everyone who is registered to vote. If we did the latter, we would get the true percentage of people who, at that moment, are likely to vote for Holmes. This is impractical not least because it's time consuming and expensive. Therefore, we can only poll a sample of voters. If this sample is representative of all likely voters, and this means we've taken a random sample of some sort, we can draw some general conclusions about all likely voters, not just the ones we questioned.

This is where precision information is valuable. If the results of the poll indicated that Holmes was winning 52% of the vote plus or minus 1% with 90% confidence, then we would conclude that there is a 90% chance that the interval 51% to 53% includes the actual percentage who are likely to vote for him. 51% to 53% is called a confidence interval. All the values in this interval indicate that Holmes will win.

However, if it was plus or minus 3%, then the 90% confidence interval would be 49% to 55%. This range includes values below 50%, which means *not* all values indicate that Holmes will win.

Our second interval is wider than the first, so it has a lower level of precision. That is, we are less able to pinpoint Holmes' chances of winning the election with our 49% to 55% interval. The narrower the interval, the more precise the estimate.

Our conclusion about the true popularity of Holmes is not an absolute certainty. We polled only a subset of voters, not all of them so our results are educated guesses. That is why we have to report the *level* of confidence in our interval.

For our poverty estimates, the confidence level is 90%. (The U.S. government usually sets its confidence level to 90%.) The SPM estimate for 2017 is 13.9% and the 90% confidence interval is 13.6% to 14.2%. This means that there is a 90% chance that the interval 13.6% to 14.2% includes the poverty rate value we would have computed had we collected information on everyone in the country, as opposed to just the families studied in the Annual Social and Economic Supplement of the CPS. (Interestingly enough, in the U.S., unemployment rates were the first to be published with confidence intervals.)

The SPM is considered a "quasi-relative" measure, so in between an absolute and a relative one. It's considered somewhat relative, because the 33rd percentile of actual expenditures is considered as opposed to imposing a minimum budget. It is still an absolute measure because these calculations aren't done using income, only expenditures. While it is used only for informational, not official, purposes, it is helpful to paint a more nuanced picture of poverty in the U.S.

SUMMARY

The primary choice in poverty measurement is between taking an absolute versus a relative approach. The former is favored by the U.S. whereas the latter is preferred by the European Union. The Census Bureau uses an income threshold to determine whether or not a family is considered poor. The poverty rate, then, is the percentage of people living in poor families.

This income threshold was developed by Mollie Orshansky, who used information about food to construct the measure. This was the information available to her given nearly a century of USDA research. Her measure—food cost times three adjusted for inflation—is now considered woefully outdated.

The threshold is calculated at the national level and adjusted for family size and composition. It is used to calculate both national and local poverty estimates, through the Current Population Survey and the Small Area Income and Poverty Estimates program. Federal fund allocations are then made using the local poverty estimates. In addition, eligibility for government benefits is determined by comparing the national threshold to household income. Examples include Head Start, the National School Lunch Program, the Children's Health Insurance Program, and the Supplemental Nutrition Assistance Program.

More recently, the Census Bureau has begun to publish the Supplemental Poverty Measure (SPM) alongside the official measure. The SPM income threshold is calculated using actual expenditures for food, clothing, shelter, and utilities, and is adjusted to account for things like geographical differences.

FURTHER READING

Nickel and Dimed: On (Not) Getting By in America by Barbara Ehrenreich. Picador, 2011.

Ehrenreich attempts to eke out a living in a series of low-wage jobs, from waitressing to housekeeping to retail. Even in towns where the cost of living is low, she finds it difficult to earn enough—even with, at times, two jobs—to live decently and save for any future setbacks. In her humorous style, she observes that her life was cushier and healthier prior to her experiment. She finds her choices to improve her life limited by mental and physical exhaustion along with various systemic issues. Her verdict is that leaving people with no way out of poverty is not the mark of a just society.

Poverty Knowledge: Social Science, Social Policy, and the Poor in Twentieth-Century History by Alice O'Connor. Princeton University Press, 2001.

While much of this chapter has focused on history, we've really only scratched the surface. O'Connor's book goes far deeper. Of particular interest is that Johnson's War on Poverty spawned a new industry of evaluating government programs. She demonstrates that there are many things to be measured in regards to poverty, not just the poverty rate.

Automating Inequality: How High-Tech Tools Profile, Police, and Punish the Poor by Virginia Eubanks. St. Martin's Press, 2018.

This book pairs well with O'Connor's by focusing on modern case studies of welfare programs. Eubanks shows how technology is used to reduce costs and ostensibly increase the efficiency of these programs. However, these technologies lead to many ethical quandaries as "objective" algorithms try to categorize and make decisions about messy, human lives.

CHAPTER 7

Deprivation

THE WORD "POOR" evokes an image of more than just someone whose income is low. Charles Dickens equipped us with a graphic description in *Oliver Twist*: "Child as he was, he was desperate with hunger, and reckless with misery...somewhat alarmed at his own temerity: 'Please, sir, I want some more.'"[61]

Living in poverty could mean you lack indoor plumbing. It could mean you attend a school where the textbooks are fifty years old. It could even mean you need to take three buses and the subway to get to work.

This broader sense of poverty is called "deprivation." In 1980, a government-commissioned report on health inequality in the United Kingdom was published. It became known as the Black Report after its chair, Sir Douglas Black. The report concluded that health disparities were getting worse, even though healthcare was available through the National Health Service.

Given these gloomy results, the government tried to limit its impact by printing only a few copies. That attempt failed. One lasting effect of the report was piquing researchers' interests, giving rise to deprivation indices. These were used to identify regions of the country which had higher rates of disease.[154] The Townsend Material Deprivation Index, is the most famous deprivation index to arise from this era of research.

Currently, the United Kingdom publishes the Index of Multiple Deprivation which itself is a combination of several deprivation indices. In the U.S., similar types of indices are used to identify regions with a shortfall of healthcare providers or areas which would be especially vulnerable in the event of a disaster.

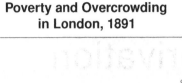

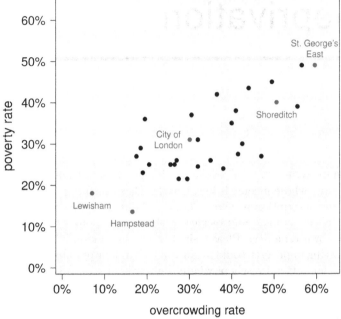

Figure 7.1 This scatterplot shows that overcrowding and poverty rates in Victorian-era London have a positive relationship. Various neighborhoods are marked including the City of London, which corresponds to the original Roman city of Londinium and is currently a business district. (Source: Graph created from table on page 567 of Charles Booth's 1893 presidential address to the Royal Statistical Society.[13])

IT'S ALL RELATIVE

Charles Booth, whom we met in the previous chapter, tried to quantify many factors potentially contributing to poverty from the age a person first marries to death rates. One of these factors was overcrowding.

Picture a family with two parents and two children. If they lived in a four-bedroom house with a living room, then everyone, if they wanted, could have their own space with one room to spare.

On the other hand, if they lived in a one-bedroom apartment with one bedroom (obviously) and a living room, then this would be two people per room, a considerably less appealing set up. The latter would be considered an overcrowded home.

People thought that having to squeeze many people into tight quarters was a marker of poverty. Charles Booth studied this claim using census data from Victorian-era London. He defined an overcrowded household as one where there were two or more people living per room or living in a lodging house. He then applied this rule to data from the 1891 Census of England to get the overcrowding rate. For thirty neighborhoods in London, he compared this rate with his own, observation-based poverty rate.[13] His results appear in Figure 7.1.

This graph is called a scatterplot. The horizontal axis of the graph displays overcrowding and the vertical one displays poverty. Each point on the plot represents a neighborhood in London.

This scatterplot shows there is a positive relationship between these two factors because, in general, as the percentage of people who live in overcrowded homes grows within a neighborhood, so does the poverty rate. Moreover, the relationship looks like it can be explained using a straight line, not a curve. (We would see a negative relationship if poverty decreased as overcrowding increased.)

In statistics, observing a straight line relationship indicates that the two factors are correlated, in this case positively correlated. To get a better idea of what that means, see Figure 7.2. Here we have four hypothetical scenarios. If Booth's graph looked like Figure 7.2A, then poverty and overcrowding would have no discernible relationship at all. This would indicate that they were uncorrelated. On the other hand, if his plot looked like Figure 7.2D, then poverty and overcrowding would have been perfectly correlated. That is, the points would form a straight line with no strays.

Booth's plot in Figure 7.1 looks like something in between Figure 7.2B and Figure 7.2C. The more the points look like they form a line, the stronger the correlation. Since our imaginary lines are sloping upwards, the correlation is positive; if the line was sloping downwards, then we would have a negative correlation. (However, if the pattern we see in our plot looks curved, not straight, then we can't use the statistical word correlation to describe the relationship.)

What we can't say is that overcrowding causes poverty or that poverty causes overcrowding. It may or may not, but our plot fails to give us any information on that front; we only know that there is a pattern for London in 1891 when we define poverty and over-crowding the way Booth does. It's possible that this correlation doesn't apply to other cities or other years of data.

It's tempting to jump from seeing a pattern to assuming a causal relationship, but two silly examples will hopefully disabuse you of that notion: It just so happens that the number of letters in the word spelled by the Scripps National Spelling Bee champion is correlated with the number of people who die each year after being bitten by a spider. Here is another one: The per capita consumption of mozzarella cheese is correlated with the number of people each year who earn a Ph.D. in civil engineering.[153] There is absolutely no reason to suspect spiders creep around spelling bees or that civil engineers are keen on mozzarella. These are just patterns that happen to have been noticed by someone.

Similarly, overcrowding and poverty are correlated, but all we can conclude from our graph is that there is a pattern, nothing else. Moreover, this pattern describes neighborhoods, not households. And so, not every home which is overcrowded is poor or vice versa. In fact, there are probably cases where people stay out of poverty by choosing to share rooms in a smaller home.

After the Black Report was published in 1980, another correlation researchers studied was between deprivation and health. Comprehensive health data was difficult to obtain in England, but living conditions were not, thanks to the census. They decided to use information about people's living conditions as a proxy for overall health needs. For example, one such index was positively correlated with depression rates.[158] After identifying deprived regions, they directed more healthcare services to them.

A FANCY SUM

Most currently used deprivation indices are summated indices. That is, we (literally) sum up information about a bunch of factors. The resulting number is the index. We could have one such index value for every, say, county in the state.

The actual index values are not particularly helpful. Sorting them from smallest to largest, however, yields a ranking from the least deprived county to the most deprived one. From year to year, we can see if this ranking shifts.

The Townsend Material Deprivation Index, the most famous summated deprivation index, was developed by the sociologist Peter Townsend in the late 1980s to identify regions in northern

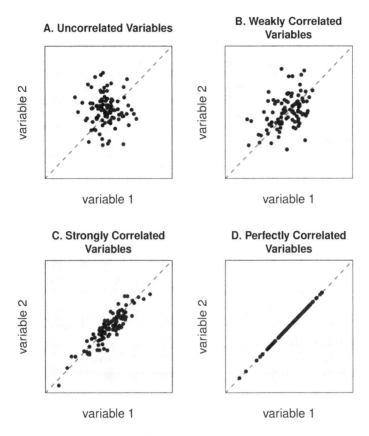

Figure 7.2 Comparing different types of relationships using hypothetical data. Correlation measures how well the points in our plot can be approximated by a straight line. In A, we really have no relationship between the two variables; all we have is a cloud of points. Both B and C show a linear relationship between the two variables, just C is stronger because the points form a clearer line. In D, we have perfect correlation in that there are no points which deviate from a straight line.

England where residents had more health problems.[154] (Townsend was also on the committee which produced the 1980 Black Report.) The index, along with a similar one invented by Brian Jarman, is the basis for many other deprivation indices, including the United Kingdom's Index of Multiple Deprivation.

Townsend, the measure's namesake, identified four variables which could act as proxies for health information:

- % of individuals who are unemployed,

- % of households who rent,

- % of households which are overcrowded,

- and % of households without a vehicle.

Townsend defined "overcrowding" as more than one person per room, which is a lower threshold than Booth's definition.

Each of these variables is defined so that a higher percentage indicates a higher level of deprivation. However, there are some value judgments here.

Being formally employed is *better* than not. Since unemployment is defined by counting people who are either employed or currently looking for a job, we aren't docking points for stay-at-home-parents.

Owning your home is *better* than renting. This presumes you are planning to live somewhere long enough that purchasing a home makes financial sense.

Living in a bigger house is *better* than living in a cramped one. We hope, of course, this larger house has indoor plumbing and electricity.

Finally, owning a car, truck, or van is *better* than relying on public transport, walking, or riding your bicycle. We will see the effects of these judgments when we look at our results.

To be able to compare our deprivation index with poverty rates, we will continue to use California and Ohio as our example states. There are 58 counties in California and 88 in Ohio. Both are populous.

California is home to Los Angeles, the second largest U.S. city, and Silicon Valley, which is known for both its unbridled tech success and its stratospheric property prices. Ohio, smaller in both population and land area, has many mid-size cities but a larger rural population. These contrasts will help highlight the pros and cons of deprivation indices.

To calculate the Townsend index, all four variables need to be collected for each county in Ohio (or California). These are available at the county level from the American Community Survey (ACS). Since some counties have few residents, we will use data combined over multiple years, from 2013 to 2017.[39]

As the section title suggests, we eventually will need to add up our four pieces of information. But not yet. Even though each variable is a percentage—and so is between 0% and 100%—they still aren't comparable. Figure 7.3A explains why.

Each line segment in Figure 7.3A corresponds to a variable in the deprivation index. The dots mark the Ohio counties with the smallest and largest values of that variable; the vertical line flags the average value.

The distance between the minimum and maximum values is called the range in statistics. It's the simplest measure of how spread out the numbers are in a data set.

Figure 7.3A shows that unemployment and overcrowding are both low for all Ohio counties and so have a narrow range. The "no vehicle" and rental variables have wider ranges, although rental has a much higher average.

The key issue is that every single county in Ohio has a rental percentage which is higher than any unemployment or overcrowded percentage. That is, the line segments do not overlap. Therefore, if we added the four percentages for a county as is, the rental component would have the largest impact on whether that county is considered deprived or not.

If we repeated this exercise with another state, a different variable may have the largest impact. This is not what we want. Rather, it would be preferable to have each component of the index have a fixed impact on the final deprivation value. The Townsend index goes further and stipulates that each variable have an equal impact on the index (i.e., equally weighted).

To solve this problem—to make the components comparable—they must be rescaled as follows:

1. Transform the values for each variable with the goal of making that variable's histogram more symmetric. An example of such a transformation is a logarithm, which we discussed in the housing chapter; another example is the square root.

2. Subtract the average of each variable from each transformed value of that variable. This step is called centering. Visually, this means we slide the line segments in Figure 7.3A leftward until the average value for each variable (the vertical bar) reaches zero. After this step, each county's centered unemployment rate, for example, is how far that county's unemployment rate is from the county average.

3. Divide each centered value by the standard deviation of the corresponding variable.

Symmetric variables are better when we are interested in averages. (Recall from the inequality chapter about what happens to the average salary of employees in a company when one employee makes a million dollars and everyone else earns far less.) Therefore, the first step sets things up so that the centering step is more useful. The second and third step combined are called *standardization* (and the resulting values are called z-scores). Let's look more closely at the third step.

Initially, we looked at the range, the distance from the smallest to the largest value for a variable, as a way to think about spread. One downside is that if there is one very large (or very small) value, compared to the others, the range will look artificially large. The same type of issue crops up with computing the average instead of the median (middle value) when we have skewed data. A single outlier can have an outsize impact on the results. (We also saw this in the employee salaries example from the inequality chapter.)

A better measure of spread, or variability, is called the standard deviation. This number tells us, on average, how far each observation is from the actual average. (Standard deviation is also affected by outliers but is more robust than the range.)

For example, if the standard deviation of overcrowding is small, then Ohio counties would have similar overcrowding percentages. At the extreme, if all counties had exactly the same overcrowding rate, then the standard deviation would be 0. That is, no variability at all. In contrast, if the standard deviation is large, then overcrowding would vary a lot across counties.

All four variables have an average of 0 after centering (step 2), and dividing by the standard deviation causes all of them to have a standard deviation of 1. The third step also has the (desired) effect of producing county values which are stripped of their units. We are left with information in standardized units, that is, the number of standard deviations the county variable is from the variable average. This allows comparisons of things that are kilograms or meters or percentages without getting bogged down by their units of measurement or large differences in magnitude across variables.

The four variables are now comparable. This is visible if we look back to Figure 7.3B which repeats the first plot using the transformed and rescaled data. Values above 3 (or -3) on the plot indicate counties that have anomalous values for that variable. In statistics, these counties would be called outliers. The largest

A. Original Variables for Ohio Counties

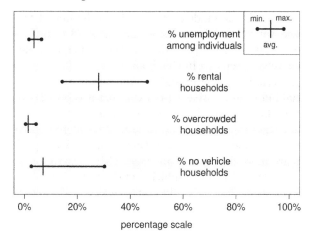

B. Transformed and Standardized Variables for Ohio Counties

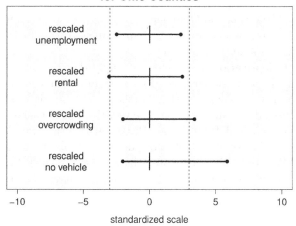

Figure 7.3 Comparing the original (plot A) and the standard-ized components (plot B) of the Townsend Material Depri-vation Index. Each horizontal segment marks the range, the minimum value to the maximum value. The vertical line marks the average percentage across the counties. Counties with val-ues beyond +3 or −3 in plot B are considered outliers. (Source: 2013–2017 American Community Survey 5-year estimates.)

outlier is Holmes County, with a standardized value of 5.88 for the "no vehicle" variable.

The "deprivation index" emerges from the sum of the four standardized variables. The index is the set of 88 sums, one for each county in Ohio. (This procedure is very different from the other indices we've discussed in this book.)

The actual deprivation index value for a county, apart from the minimal information we get from whether it is positive or negative, is not too helpful. We know that a higher unemployment or rental rate, for instance, is supposed to indicate a more deprived county. Therefore, at most we can say that counties with positive index values are more deprived than those with negative ones.

A more valuable interpretation of the index is to compare levels across counties. Figure 7.4 illustrates this type of comparison. Each vertical line represents the index level for a county sorted from smallest to largest.

In California, we can see that Sierra County is by far the least deprived and San Francisco County the most. Similarly, Noble County is the least deprived in Ohio and Holmes County the most. As the California and Ohio deprivation indices were calculated separately, we can't compare the San Francisco County index value with the Holmes County one.

Our deprivation index does not imply that everyone in Holmes County is going hungry nor does it signify that everyone in Noble County employs a butler. Furthermore, since it is a relational measure, all of California could be wealthy, but households in some counties can (only!) afford one BMW rather than two. And so the single BMW counties look more deprived than the double BMW ones. We could also encounter the reverse scenario. Perhaps the state's residents are poor, but some counties have families who can afford to eat only one meal a day whereas others can eat two. To help provide context for our deprivation index, let's bring back the poverty measure from the previous chapter.

POVERTY VS. DEPRIVATION

We started this chapter by wondering whether poverty—as measured with an income threshold—was too narrow a concept. However, one advantage of such a measure is it can be stated without a lot of messy details. We can say 15% of the county is poor and people will understand what we mean.

Townsend Material Deprivation Index

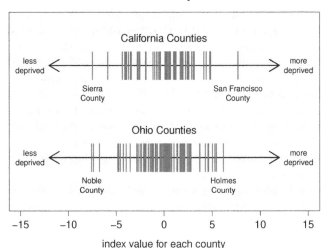

Figure 7.4 Each vertical line (blue) marks the deprivation value for a county in either California or Ohio. Higher values indicate more deprivation, relative to the other counties in the corresponding state. The least and most deprived counties in each state are noted. (Source: 2013–2017 American Community Survey 5-year estimates.)

The deprivation value for a county, in contrast, has a very technical definition and can only be interpreted relative to other counties. Accordingly, it is harder to communicate to the public.

The debate, then, is whether going through all of this effort is worth it for a measure which is difficult to explain to others. We want to know whether we really get different information about a county when we use deprivation instead of poverty.

In statistical terms, this means we want to check whether poverty and deprivation, as we've measured them, are correlated or at least show some relationship. To make such a comparison, we have to compare both measures at the county level.

The official poverty rate is national, but county-level estimates of poverty are available through the Small Area Income and Poverty Estimates (SAIPE) program run by the Census Bureau.

SAIPE applies the national poverty income threshold to ACS data to get local—that is, "small area"—estimates.[38]

To calculate our deprivation index, we used ACS estimates computed using data from 2013 to 2017; to obtain reasonably comparable poverty values for counties, we will average the SAIPE poverty estimates over the same set of years. This produces a lot of numbers: $58 + 58 + 88 + 88 = 292$ pieces of information about two states and two measures.

Since deprivation indices are interpreted by ranking the values, we could do the same with the poverty rates. That way we could figure out whether counties have similar rankings, despite the measure used. Looking at the rankings, however, still gives us 292 pieces of information to process.

To simplify things, instead of ranking from 1 to 88 in Ohio, we can divide our ranks into quintiles. This means the ranks are split into five groups (the "quint" part of the quintile).

The bottom 20% of poverty rankings makes up the first quintile. These would be the least poor counties in Ohio. The top 20% of ranks would be the fifth quintile, representing the poorest counties. (We used a similar concept in the inequality chapter, but we chopped up our data into ten groups called deciles, instead of five.) We could then draw a map, with each county shaded by quintile.

Figures 7.5 and 7.6 contain two maps each. The top map shows poverty rates and the bottom one deprivation. The counties with no shading represent the counties with deprivation or poverty ranks in the bottom quintile, meaning they are the least deprived or the least poor. Counties shaded the darkest gray represent those in the top quintile, indicating that they are the most deprived or the poorest. (County borders have been omitted on the maps so that they are easier to interpret.)

If the poverty and deprivation ranks were the same, then both maps would look exactly the same. Each county would have the same color. Clearly that is not the case.

Translating our deprivation results in Figure 7.4 onto our maps, San Francisco County in California would be shaded dark gray, the color of the most deprived areas, or the fifth quintile. However, in terms of poverty rates, it's only in the second quintile. Our poverty data is saying San Francisco County is not very poor relative to other counties in California, but our deprivation data is telling us the opposite.

If we switch to the map of Ohio, we have two maps which look much more similar, indicating that the poverty and deprivation

California Poverty Rates Ranked by County

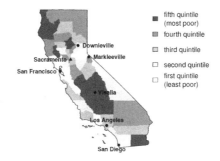

California Townsend Material Deprivation Index Values Ranked by County

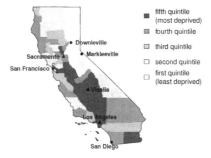

Figure 7.5 Poverty and deprivation levels by quintile (bottom 20% to top 20%) are shown for California with major cities marked; county borders have been omitted for clarity. San Francisco County is the most deprived county in California, whereas nearby San Mateo County is the least poor. Visalia, county seat of Tulare County, is in the poorest county. Downieville is the county seat of Sierra County, the least deprived county. Markleeville is the county seat of Alpine County, the least populous county in California and one of three counties in the state which is completely rural. (Sources: 2013–2017 Small Area Income and Poverty Estimates program; 2013–2017 American Community Survey 5-year estimates; 2017 Population Estimates Program; Census Bureau, Geography Division.)

Ohio Poverty Rates Ranked by County

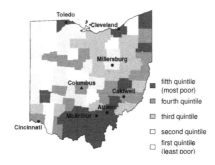

Ohio Townsend Material Deprivation Index Values Ranked by County

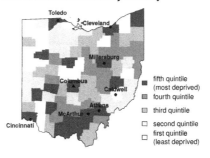

Figure 7.6 Poverty and deprivation levels by quintile (bottom 20% to top 20%) are shown for Ohio with major cities marked; county borders have been omitted for clarity. McArthur is the county seat of Vinton County, the least populous in Ohio and the only completely rural county. Millersburg is the county seat of Holmes County, the most deprived county in Ohio; Athens County is the poorest. Delaware County, which incorporates a small portion of north Columbus (which is primarily in Franklin County) is the second least deprived and the least poor. Noble County is the least deprived with Caldwell as its county seat. (Sources: 2013–2017 Small Area Income and Poverty Estimates program; 2013–2017 American Community Survey 5-year estimates; 2017 Population Estimates Program; Census Bureau, Geography Division.)

rankings are more alike for Ohio than they were for California. For example, the southern part of the state is in the fifth quintile (dark gray) for both measures.

We saw earlier that Noble County was the least deprived in Ohio, with Delaware County as a close second; both are white on the map. Delaware is also the least poor county in the state. This match between poverty and deprivation ranks seems like a point in favor of deprivation indices. However, Noble County is in the fourth quintile in terms of poverty (e.g., in the bottom half), which doesn't match at all.

On the other hand, the most deprived county in Ohio is Holmes of which Millersburg is the county seat. The same county on the poverty map is light gray, however, indicating that it is in the second quintile. Therefore, it has a poverty rate on the lower end among Ohio counties. This switch is just like the one we saw for San Francisco and the reverse of what we saw for Noble.

A second way of presenting our two measures is by using a scatterplot, like those in Figure 7.7. Here, the horizontal axis shows the deprivation index whereas the vertical axis shows the poverty rate. Each point represents a county.

By using a scatterplot instead of a map to show our results, we lose geographical context, but gain information about correlation. California counties create a loose blob in Figure 7.7A. For Ohio, however, we can draw a clear, upward sloping line. This tells us that the two variables are more strongly correlated for Ohio than for California. (To determine why this is true would require far more analysis than we can do here.)

We can also see here San Francisco County is highly deprived, but not very (relatively speaking) poor. Holmes County also sticks out in the Ohio plot. It too has a high deprivation index value, but not a correspondingly high poverty rate.

As unlikely as it seems, San Francisco County and Holmes County are closely linked. We will solve this mystery in the next section.

SKYSCRAPERS AND SILOS

Urban lifestyles differ from rural ones. Types of professions, commute times, even access to schools and hospitals can vary wildly. These differences, unfortunately, can impact interpretations of deprivation indices.

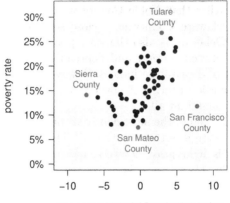

A. Poverty Rate vs. Deprivation Level
for California Counties

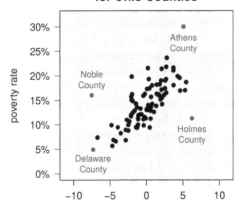

B. Poverty Rate vs. Deprivation Level
for Ohio Counties

Figure 7.7 These two scatterplots show that the linear relationship between poverty and deprivation is stronger for Ohio than for California. Notable counties are marked in blue. (Sources: 2013–2017 Small Area Income and Poverty Estimates program; 2013–2017 American Community Survey 5-year estimates.)

The histograms in Figure 7.8 show the percentage of rural residents in each county.[31] The top graph tells us that most California counties have more than 50% of their residents living in an urban area. That means only a few counties have a majority rural population and so the data is considered right-skewed. Ohio, on the other hand, has a more symmetric distribution. That means roughly half the counties have a majority urban population and the other half, a majority rural population.

Both California and Ohio have more urban residents than rural ones. However, San Francisco in California is the only county in either state with only urban residents. On the flip side, there are four completely rural counties: Vinton in Ohio along with Alpine, Mariposa, and Trinity in California. Part of the reason why there are so few residents is that large tracts of land within them are forests and parks.

This urban-rural data can be connected to the four deprivation index variables. In Figure 7.9, the first column of scatterplots represents counties in California; the second represents Ohio. On the horizontal axis of each plot, the percentage of rural residents is given. On the vertical axis, the deprivation index variables are shown. Each dot on the scatterplots represents a single county.

The top row displays unemployment rates. For California, if we drew a line representing the way the points cluster on the graph, the trend would be flat. That is, the correlation between unemployment and percentage of rural residents at the county level is very low. For Ohio, we see a gentle curve, indicating slightly higher levels of unemployment for extremely urban and extremely rural counties. (Remember, we can only be sure this pattern applies to these states during the 2013–2017 time period.)

Rental rates in the second row show a negative trend for both states (a negative correlation). Counties with more rural residents tend to also be less likely to rent their homes. This pattern is one of the reasons why the Supplemental Poverty Measure separates households into categories depending on whether they rent or own their homes. If you own your home and don't have a mortgage, you probably need less money to survive.

If we look at the third row in Figure 7.9, we have contrasting plots. At first glance, it seems like as counties in California become more rural, overcrowding becomes less of an issue. Perhaps this makes sense if we expect rural areas to be more spacious—rolling

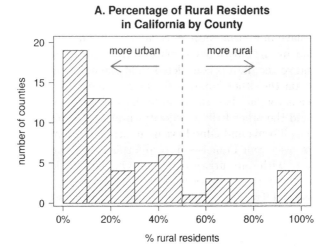

A. Percentage of Rural Residents
in California by County

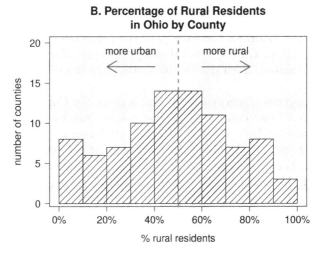

B. Percentage of Rural Residents
in Ohio by County

Figure 7.8 These histograms show the distribution of counties based on how rural they are. San Francisco County in California is the only county in either state where the entire population is classified as urban. Vinton County is the only Ohio county which is completely rural. However, California has three such counties: Alpine County, Mariposa County, and Trinity County. National forests or parks cover large parts of these four counties. (Source: 2010 Decennial Census.)

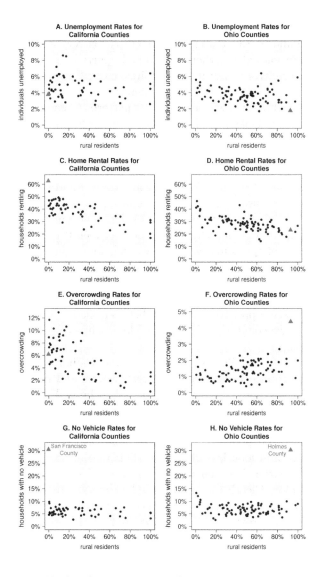

Figure 7.9 Each deprivation index component is graphed against the percentage of rural residents. San Francisco County (left, California) and Holmes County (right, Ohio) are marked as blue triangles. Both counties have many residents without vehicles. (Sources: 2013–2017 American Community Survey 5-year estimates; 2010 Decennial Census.)

hills, flat plains—and where people can build more rooms in their homes. Land in San Francisco, in contrast, is very expensive and people are packed together in cramped apartments. In any case, this is a negative trend; it looks a little curved, so we should not use the statistical term correlation here.

In Ohio, however, we see a different pattern. As counties become more rural, it looks like the rate of overcrowding increases. This could be because rural counties are poorer in Ohio and so residents can only afford to build smaller homes.

If we look more closely at the vertical axis, however, we get a more nuanced picture. The vertical axis in Figure 7.9E, which looks at overcrowding in California, starts from 0% and ends a bit above 12%, which is a wide range. On the other hand, the vertical axis in Figure 7.9F for Ohio only goes between 0% and 5% with all but one of the counties below 3%. So, we might have a trend for Ohio counties, but it's pretty minor.

To see if poverty and overcrowding are even related, we can compare them like Charles Booth did in London (Figure 7.1). His graph showed a positive correlation between these variables. It was clear that we could draw an upward sloping line to represent that relationship.

If we made similar plots for Ohio and California, we would learn two things. First, both the overcrowding and poverty rates are much lower now than they appeared to be in Victorian London. (There is a bit of handwaving here since Booth defined both variables differently in his analysis.)

Second, the points would be far more dispersed than in his scatterplot and look less like a line. This means we would have a weak correlation between variables compared to a strong one in Booth's plot. Clearly, we would need to investigate beyond just poverty rates to determine why Ohio and California differ.

In the final row of Figure 7.9, we look at the relationship between not owning a vehicle and how rural the county is. Both states look relatively similar and have a flat trend. Both also have one point (shown as a blue triangle) which is much farther away from the others. That is, these counties are outliers: Around 30% of their households survive without owning a car, truck, or van.

In California, that triangle represents San Francisco County, home to a variety of public transit options. In Ohio, the triangle represents Holmes County and is almost completely rural. And why don't they have vehicles? Holmes County is home (pun intended) to one of the largest Amish communities in the U.S. They use a horse and buggy to travel, not cars. Therefore, they are counted as *not* owning vehicles.

What is striking about this example is that in neither case would an observer consider households in these counties deprived when it comes to transport. Sure, it's nice to have access to a car, but you can get around perfectly well in both places without one. Moreover, in San Francisco, having a vehicle would probably be more of a marker of affluence than of deprivation.

Consequently, the vehicle variable doesn't really apply to these counties, but since they are part of their respective states, they stick out on this dimension.

Both San Francisco and Holmes are marked with a blue triangle in all of the graphs in Figure 7.9. Apart from perhaps overcrowding in Holmes, neither county sticks out among the other dimensions of Townsend's index.

However, the "no vehicle" dimension is so different that it catapults both counties into the unfortunate honor of being the most deprived county in their respective states. The poverty rates, in contrast, place both in the second quintile.. That means they have poverty rates lower than most of the other counties in the state. The deprivation index says these counties are in crisis, but the poverty rates say the opposite.

This is a major downside to deprivation indices. If we combine heterogenous counties to create our index, the variables we choose may be relevant to some counties but not others. Counties have to be roughly comparable in order for the deprivation index to be meaningful. Our San Francisco and Holmes County results demonstrate what happens when we ignore that principle.

EVEN FANCIER SUMS

The Townsend Material Deprivation Index acted as a template for subsequent indices. Researchers proposed alternative variables, added new ones, or weighted the factors differently, giving more importance to some variables than to others.

For example, the Index of Multiple Deprivation, computed in the United Kingdom, has several deprivation indices within it representing "domains" like crime, employment, and education. These individual indices are then combined to get the final index. This is why the name of the index includes the word "multiple."[102]

Here is a list of just some of the factors included in deprivation indices from the United Kingdom, South Africa, New Zealand, and Namibia:[7, 102, 111, 112]

distance to supermarket	no trash removal service
traffic accidents	secondary school absence
no internet access	housing affordability
single parent family	welfare benefits
air quality	literacy
crime rates	no electricity
homelessness	no television
distance to doctor	mood and anxiety disorders

The longer the list of factors, the more complicated the index and the harder it is to interpret. Furthermore, on the practical front, you must be able to assemble all of those variables each time you want to calculate the index in the future. Losing even one variable produces a different index. Consequently, balancing practicality, interpretability, and relevance is a challenging task.

Within the U.S., there are a few summated indices in use. The Health Resources & Services Administration creates the Index of Medical Underservice and it also uses summated indices to assign the designation Health Professional Shortage Area (similar to how Townsend's original index was used). In addition, the Social Vulnerability Index, published by the Centers for Disease Control and Prevention, uses information to identify regions which may need more assistance after disasters such as hurricanes.

SUMMARY

Poverty measures focus on income whereas deprivation measures are more holistic. Given this more nuanced approach, deprivation measures are gaining steam as a supplement to poverty rates.

Summated indices, like the Townsend Material Deprivation Index, are a common way to combine information about multiple factors, like unemployment and rental rates, into a single number. They are computed using data from several regions (like counties) producing one index value per region. These values are then ranked to determine the least deprived region to the most deprived one.

Ranking makes deprivation indices a relative measure; that is, we evaluate how relatively deprived a region is by comparing it to its neighbor. This can be limiting. For example, calculating the index for all counties in Ohio separately from all counties in

California means that we can't compare Ohio with California. It also makes it tough to see how well Franklin County in Ohio is doing from year to year apart from looking at how its rank changes. We can't tell, in an absolute sense, whether the county has become less deprived, only that it is less deprived than another county.

Furthermore, just as not all people in deprived areas are indigent, not all people in affluent areas are in good shape. These indices are general statements about a region and so shouldn't be applied to individual people.

Which variables to include is highly contextual. Some factors may be relevant in rural areas, but not urban ones and should vary across countries. This can make the interpretation of the index difficult or at times inadvisable when computed for a heterogenous group of areas. Therefore the selection of the areas is just as important as which variables are chosen.

FURTHER READING

The Great Escape: Health, Wealth, and the Origins of Inequality by Angus Deaton. Princeton University Press, 2013.

This book explores the relationships among income, health, and happiness. It includes excellent discussions about what can and cannot be inferred from measures designed to describe poverty and well-being.

Hillbilly Elegy: A Memoir of a Family and Culture in Crisis by J.D. Vance. HarperCollins Publishers, 2016.

This memoir gives context to deprivation measurement. Through his experience of growing up in small-town Ohio and eastern Kentucky, Vance describes how a combination of factors—jobs, home ownership, sense of community, access to education, and so forth—contribute to deprivation. This case study at its core suggests that a simple poverty line measure fails to capture the complexity behind the failure or success of rural communities.

Affluence Without Abundance: The Disappearing World of the Bushmen by James Suzman. Bloomsbury USA, 2017.

The idea that someone is considered deprived in a society is entirely dependent on what that society deems as its requirements. The goals of every society are different, therefore the definition of what it is to be deprived must also vary. This book provides an illustration of what happens when the goals of one society are applied to another. To make his argument, Suzman's ethnography focuses on the effects of colonialism and governmental policy on hunter-gatherer tribes in modern Namibia.

CHAPTER 8

Postscript

During a Congressional session about the first U.S. census, James Madison, noted, "I take it, sir, that in order to accommodate our laws to the real situation of our constituents, we ought to be acquainted with that situation."[98]

Madison was right. Collecting and publishing data about the inhabitants of a society is crucial to improving it. That this book could even be written is a testament to the notion of improvement through data.

However, despite these efforts at dissemination and transparency, many people can only guess, for example, what the unemployment rate is. Few know how it's measured. Moreover, many have little trust in official statistics and the agencies which produce them.

Whether or not you think unemployment is too high depends on what you think the unemployment rate actually is. In 2018, marketing research firm Ipsos asked Americans, "Out of every 100 people of working age in the United States, about how many do you think are unemployed and looking for work?" The average answer was 22 when in actuality it was only 4 people out of every 100.[141] This is a large gap!

Your answer to this question is also based on what you think the working age is, what it means to be unemployed, and what counts as "looking for work." These are questions about measurement. Hopefully this book helped with that.

Furthermore, accepting the published statistic requires two things: faith in the institution constructing the statistic and trust in the respondents of the surveys used to produce that statistic.

To ensure the latter, guaranteeing the confidentiality of responses to surveys is critical.

The Census Bureau, for example, has many ways to mask the identity of responders such as publishing data only at higher levels of aggregation or adding noise to the data. Moreover, laws exist to restrict access to only those with authorization.

The necessity of guarding respondents' privacy was highlighted during World War II. Census records were used to find and imprison people of Japanese descent—many of them American citizens—in internment camps. This was a direct result of a regrettable act passed in 1942 which suspended the usual confidentiality rules.[5] (These rules were restored after the war and remain in place today.)

Ironically, acceptance of statistics leads to its own set of problems. These can be divided into two broad issues—first the potential misappropriation of statistics for use in policy recommendations, and second, the tendency for measures to ossify once they begin to play a central role in government policy.

Even accounting for these problems, there is no doubt, as you've seen in these chapters, that measuring society has enhanced our lives.

We end with one, final statistic, presented in two ways: The 2010 census cost $12.3 billion. This is a lot of money, and part of the cost was because people ignored their census forms and had to be personally contacted. This amount, however, was spent over a decade of preparation and comes down to only about $92 per household.[79] That really isn't much at all.

FURTHER READING

The Politics of Numbers edited by William Alonso and Paul Starr. Russell Sage Foundation, 1987.

> The world has changed significantly since this book was written, but its points are still relevant. The various authors of this edited volume examine a wide set of statistics produced by the U.S. government covering topics about income to ethnicity to voting patterns in order to describe how politics affect measurement. Throughout, they consider what it means for the public to trust the official numbers.

The Tyranny of Metrics by Jerry Z. Muller. Princeton University Press, 2018.

This book focuses on measurement, its history, and its consequences. Muller deploys the term "metric fixation" which means using a only few statistics to describe and incentivize a complex organization. Within government, statistics like unemployment and inflation fall into this trap. These numbers, along with a few others, like GDP, were not intended to completely describe a vast, interconnected, and global economy, but they eventually were used that way.

"'In order that they might rest their arguments on facts': The vital role of government-collected data" by Nicholas Eberstadt, Ryan Nunn, Diane Whitmore Schanzenbach, and Michael R. Strain. The Hamilton Project at the Brookings Institution and the American Enterprise Institute, March 2017.

On the (hopefully) off chance this book hasn't made the case for the importance of official statistics, perhaps this report will. The authors show how businesses, policy makers, and families make use of this vast array of government-collected, but publicly available information. They argue that such data is critical for a modern nation to succeed.

Glossary

Listed here are definitions for statistical terms and graphs along with descriptions of the major, publicly available data sources used in this book.

American Community Survey (ACS): This survey is conducted by the Census Bureau and collects data on social, housing, economic, and demographic characteristics of the U.S. population. The results are published annually. For small geographic areas, like school districts or census tracts, estimates are computed from data combined across several years. Funding for many federal and state programs are distributed based on the results of this survey.

American Housing Survey (AHS): This survey is conducted by the Census Bureau to collect information about the quantity and quality of housing. The U.S. Department of Housing and Urban Development (HUD) uses this data to develop its policies.

bar graph: A way to visualize qualitative data. Each bar represents one category and the height of the bar specifies a numerical value like the frequency of that category (see Figure 4.5B on page 62 about housing) or some other numerical quantity (see Figure 6.6 on page 115 about average expenditures by region).

Bureau of Labor Statistics (BLS): Part of the U.S. Department of Labor and the second largest federal statistical agency. This bureau is in charge of labor statistics and other economic statistics, including unemployment and the Consumer Price Index (used to measure inflation).

Census Bureau: Part of the U.S. Department of Commerce and the largest federal statistical agency. It administers the decennial census along with many other statistical surveys, including ACS, AHS, and CPS. It also runs PEP, SAIPE, and additional research programs to improve data collection and estimation procedures.

Early in U.S. history, the agency would exist only during decennial census activities. In 1902, Congress made the Census Office permanent and eventually renamed it the Census Bureau.

confidence interval: The most commonly encountered confidence intervals are probably those associated with election polls. Usually something like, "Candidate A will win 52% of the vote plus or minus 1 percentage point," is reported. The "plus or minus 1" part is called the margin of error and the range 51% to 53% is the resulting confidence interval based on the statistic 52% (52−1 to 52 + 1). The "confidence" part of a confidence interval refers to how certain you are that the interval includes the actual value. (In this example, the "actual value" is the percentage planning to vote for Candidate A if you surveyed *all* potential voters, not just those contacted in the poll.) Of course we want to be 100% sure, but the only way to be that confident is to include every possible percentage in our interval. (Again, for this example, the 100% interval would then be 0% to 100%.) In practice, 90%, 95%, and 99% confidence intervals are the most common. Wanting to be more confident results in wider intervals (the 100% interval is just the most extreme version of this principle).

Consumer Expenditure (CE) Survey: This survey is conducted by the Census Bureau on behalf of BLS. It consists of two separate surveys: the Interview Survey and the Diary Survey. Both are used to obtain information about household income and expenditures and the results are used in Consumer Price Index (CPI) calculations. The Census Bureau also uses it to calculate poverty thresholds for the Supplemental Poverty Measure (SPM), an alternative to the official poverty measure.

correlation: This term is often used to signify that two quantities are related. For example, people's heights and weights are correlated. That should sound reasonable since taller people tend to weigh more. Correlation is also a technical term in statistics which indicates that not only do two variables have a relationship, that relationship is linear. That is, if we drew a scatterplot, the best way to describe the pattern on the graph is with a straight line as opposed to a curved one. Two things can be correlated, but that tells you nothing about whether one causes the other. See Figure 7.2 on page 131 in the chapter on deprivation for an example.

Current Population Survey (CPS): This survey is conducted by the Census Bureau and is the source of unemployment (published by BLS) and poverty rate estimates. Additional data on topics like school enrollment and health insurance coverage is collected on a more ad hoc basis through CPS, including in the Annual Social and Economic Supplement (ASEC). The ASEC is used to calculate the Supplemental Poverty Measure (SPM), an alternative to the official poverty measure, by the Census Bureau.

decennial census: A full count of the population—a census—is required every ten years by the U.S. Constitution (Article I, Section 2). The results are primarily used to decide the number of members each state can send to the House of Representatives, a branch of Congress. This process is called apportionment. The first census took place in 1790 during President George Washington's administration. It is currently conducted by the Census Bureau.

geometric mean: Multiply a set of n numbers and then take the nth root. For example, the geometric mean of 4 and 9 is the square root (since $n = 2$) of 4 times 9, or the square root of 36, which is 6. This is an alternative to the usual average (or arithmetic mean) and is frequently used when you are interested in growth rates of things like prices.

histogram: A way to visualize quantitative data such as household income or age. It is essentially a bar graph for quantitative, as opposed to qualitative, data. Figure 4.5A on page 62 from the housing chapter is an example of a histogram made from the construction year of homes in San Diego, California. To make this graph, the time span from the earliest to most recent construction year is chopped into smaller periods. Those periods are the widths of each bar. The height of each bar is the number of homes whose construction year is in the corresponding range.

mean: Technical term for "average;" also called an arithmetic mean. For example, the mean of 4 and 9 is the sum of 4 and 9 divided by 2 (since there are two numbers), which equals 6.5. It is a measure of the center of a data set.

median: Like the mean, the median is a way to measure the center of a data set. An advantage of the median is that it is more robust than the mean (see robust). It is computed as follows: Order a set of numbers from smallest to largest and select the number in the middle. This value is called the median. It represents the 50th

percentile (see percentiles and quantiles) because roughly half the data is above the median and half is below.

National Bureau of Economic Research (NBER): A private organization which is nonpartisan and nonprofit. The researchers affiliated with NBER study business cycles, the impact of governmental policies, and factors contributing to economic growth. They also identify recessionary periods in the U.S. economy.

official statistic: A statistic published by a government or other public entity for informational purposes.

outlier: A piece of data which is very different from the others.

percentiles and quantiles: The 25th percentile (or the 0.25 quantile) for income, for example, is the income level at which 25% of the people earn at most that amount. The 50th percentile (or 0.5 quantile) is called the median.

percent change: The quantity (new value − old value)/old value multiplied by 100. This gives us the percent increase (if positive) or decrease (if negative) of the new value in relation to the old one.

population: In short, everyone. However, who counts as "everyone" depends on the goal. In the decennial census, the goal is to count everyone who lives in the U.S. On the other hand, for U3 unemployment, the population is everyone considered to be in the labor force, as opposed to all adults.

Population Estimates Program (PEP): The goal of this Census Bureau program is to estimate the size of the U.S. population between decennial censuses. This population estimate is then used by other federal surveys to ensure consistency of estimates across surveys. That is, all surveys are producing estimates based on a common population size.

price relative: The ratio of one price to another price.

ratio statistic: This type of statistic is computed by dividing two numbers which, themselves, are statistics. For instance, the unemployment rate is calculated by the ratio of the number of unemployed people to those in the labor force. Both parts of the ratio have to be estimated to get the final unemployment rate. This is because among the people who are surveyed, only some are considered in the labor force, and fewer are considered unemployed.

robust: A statistic which is isn't heavily impacted by outliers.

sample: A census is an expensive and time-consuming enterprise. Therefore, most of the time only a subset of the population is studied. This subset is called a sample and is used to infer characteristics about the population. To be able to do so, the sample must be collected using statistical methods which incorporate randomness into the selection process.

sampling frame: A list of all people (or items, companies, etc.) from which a sample is selected. This list is intended to enumerate everyone in the population. Mistakes in this list are called coverage errors and result in inaccuracies in the statistics computed from that sample. Examples of coverage errors are people listed twice in the sampling frame or people who are not listed at all.

scatterplot: A type of graph which shows the relationship between two numerical quantities. Figure 7.1 on page 128 in the deprivation chapter provides a typical example. Each dot on the plot represents a neighborhood in London about which two pieces of information are displayed. On the horizontal axis, we can find the percentage of overcrowded homes in that neighborhood; on the vertical axis, the corresponding poverty rate. Scatterplots are often used to visually assess correlation.

seasonality: Some patterns in time series data are cyclical—or seasonal—like the Christmas shopping rush. Such effects often make it difficult to determine whether changes in a measure are due to underlying shifts or simply because it's a certain time of the year. Therefore, statistical techniques called "seasonal adjustment" are often applied to time series data to obtain a series which is easier to interpret. Figure 2.1A on page 9 shows an example of seasonal adjustment for the labor force participation rate.

skew: This term describes a certain shape data can take. Skewness occurs when most of the data is clustered together but there are a few observations which stretch far larger than that cluster (skew to the right) or stretch far lower than that cluster (skew to the left). It is easiest to detect this property with a histogram. Figure 3.7E on page 43 is skewed to the right; Figure 4.5A on page 62 is is skewed to the left. Figure 3.7C is an example of data with no skew at all. That is, it's symmetric.

Small Area Income and Poverty Estimates (SAIPE) program: This program is run by the Census Bureau. It combines data from ACS and other sources to calculate assorted local estimates, including local poverty rates. These results are used by governments at various levels to allocate funds.

standard deviation: This number tells you how close, in general, the values used to calculate the mean (average) are to that mean. A small standard deviation indicates the numbers are clustered around the mean, a large standard deviation signifies the reverse. Often, both the mean and standard deviation are reported together, which provides more complete information about the data: where the data are clustered (the mean) and how close those data are to that mean (the standard deviation).

standardization: Compute the average (mean) and standard deviation of your data. Then, for each observation, subtract that average value and then divide by that standard deviation. The result is a standardized observation which tells you how many standard deviations the original observation is from the average. For example, if the standardized value is zero, then the original observation is exactly equal to the average; that is, zero standard deviations away. The farther away the standardized value is from zero, the farther away that particular observation is from the average. Standardized values larger than three (or -3) are often considered outliers. The Townsend Material Deprivation Index in the chapter on deprivation uses standardization.

statistic: Statistics, like graphs, are a way to summarize and describe large quantities of information (i.e., data). In its technical sense, a statistic is a number calculated using data from a sample. This definition includes many kinds of numbers. For example, the maximum value in the data is a statistic; means, medians, and standard deviations are statistics too. In a more colloquial sense, the word "statistic" is used for any number calculated from a sample or a census—basically any number calculated from data. Finally, in its plural form, "statistics" also stands for a field of study encompassing collecting, organizing, analyzing, and presenting data.

time series: The poverty rate for 2019 is a static piece of information. If the rate was listed for every year from 2000 to 2019, we would have a time series. Such data allow for a quantity (like the poverty rate or a house price index) to be tracked over time.

Figure 6.3 on page 105, which shows the poverty rate from 1959 to 2017, is a visual example of time series data.

World Inequality Database (WID.world): Every country has its own way of defining inequality and counts income, taxes, welfare payments, and so forth differently as well. This variation makes it difficult to compare inequality and other economic statistics. The researchers who maintain and grow WID.world have developed a way to apply the same definitions across all countries, making cross-country comparisons possible. Generating these estimates isn't easy: For the U.S., researchers had to access and organize records from the Federal Reserve Board, the IRS and the U.S. Census Bureau, among other organizations for each year. Thomas Piketty, whom we met in the inequality chapter, is one of the co-directors of WID.world.

Bibliography

[1] *All graphs were created in R, in part with packages written by various authors: blsAPI, gdata, lubridate, maptools, mvtnorm, openxlsx, plotrix, readxl, rgdal, rgeos, rjson, tidyverse, tmap, tmaptools.* URL: https://cran.r-project.org/.

[2] B. Alexander. *Glass House: The 1% Economy and the Shattering of the All-American Town.* St. Martin's Press, 2017.

[3] W. Alonso and P. Starr, editors. *The Politics of Numbers.* Essays for the National Committee for Research on the 1980 Census. Russell Sage Foundation, 1987.

[4] American Federation of Labor and Congress of Industrial Organizations. *Executive Paywatch*, 2015 (used with permission). URL: https://aflcio.org/paywatch.

[5] M. Anderson. *The American Census: A Social History, 2nd ed.* Yale University Press, 2015.

[6] The Associated Press. Wall St.'s bronze bull moves 2 blocks south. *The New York Times*, December 20, 1989.

[7] J. Atkinson, C. Salmond, and P. Crampton. *NZDep2013 Index of Deprivation,* 2014.

[8] W.O. Atwater. Foods: Nutritive Value and Cost. *U.S. Department of Agriculture Farmers' Bulletin No. 23,* 1894.

[9] E. Badger. When the (empty) apartment next door is owned by an oligarch. *The New York Times*, July 21, 2017.

[10] M.J. Bailey, R.F. Muth, and H.O. Nourse. A regression method for real estate price index construction. *Journal of the American Statistical Association*, 58(304):933–942, 1963.

[11] J. Bates. Survey cites four California banks with possibly risky realty loans. *Los Angeles Times*, December 30, 1989.

[12] R.M. Blank. Presidential address: How to improve poverty measurement in the United States. *Journal of Policy Analysis and Management*, 27(2):233–254, 2008.

[13] C. Booth. Life and labour of the people in London: First results of an inquiry based on the 1891 census. Opening address of Charles Booth, Esq., President of the Royal Statistical Society. Session 1893–94. *Journal of the Royal Statistical Society*, 56(4):557–593, 1893.

[14] A.L. Bowley. Address to the Economic Science and Statistics Section of the British Association for the Advancement of Science, York. *Journal of the Royal Statistical Society*, 69(3):540–558, 1906.

[15] U.S. Bureau of Economic Analysis. URL: https://www.bea.gov.

[16] U.S. Bureau of Labor Statistics. URL: https://www.bls.gov.

[17] U.S. Bureau of Labor Statistics. *Handbook of Methods.* URL: https://www.bls.gov/opub/hom/.

[18] U.S. Bureau of Labor Statistics. Series IDs: APU0000711111, APU0000711211, CUSR0000SA0, CUSR0000SA0L1E, CUSR0000SAF1, CUUR0000SA0, CUUR0000SEEB01, CUUR0000SETB01, CUUR0000SETG01, CUUR0000SEEE01, CUSR0000SA0E. *Databases: All Urban Consumers, Average Price Data.* URL: https://www.bls.gov/data/#prices.

[19] U.S. Bureau of Labor Statistics. Table A-1: Employment Status of the Civilian Population by Sex and Age; Table A-8: Employed Persons by Class of Worker and Part-Time Status; Table A-15: Alternative Measures of Labor Underutilization; Table A-16: Persons Not in the Labor Force and Multiple Jobholders by Sex, Not Seasonally Adjusted. *Current Population Survey.*

[20] U.S. Bureau of Labor Statistics. Cross-tabulated experimental tables: Region of residence by income before taxes; Size of consumer unit by income before taxes. *Consumer Expenditure Surveys*, 2016–2017. URL: https://www.bls.gov/cex/.

[21] U.S. Bureau of Labor Statistics. Cost of living in North Atlantic shipbuilding districts. *Monthly Labor Review*, 7:352–355, August 1918.

[22] U.S. Bureau of Labor Statistics. Archived Relative Importance of Components in the Consumer Price Indexes, Table 1: U.S. City Average Using 2015–2016 Weights. December 2017.

[23] U.S. Bureau of Labor Statistics. Prices and cost of living. *Monthly Labor Review*, 12:260–317, February 1921.

[24] U.S. Bureau of Labor Statistics. Table 11-1011: Occupational Employment and Wages, Chief Executives. *Occupational Employment Statistics*, May 2015.

[25] U.S. Bureau of Labor Statistics. *The Employment Situation—April 2019.* May 2019.

[26] U.S. Bureau of Labor Statistics. Retail prices of food in the United States. *Monthly Labor Review*, 3:46, September 1915.

[27] U.S. Bureau of the Census. *Fifteenth Census of the United States: 1930–Unemployment, Volume II*, 1931.

[28] D. Card. Origins of the unemployment rate: The lasting legacy of measurement without theory. *Prepared for the 2011 Meetings of the American Economic Association*, 2011.

[29] J.A. Caswell and A.L. Yaktine, editors. *Supplemental Nutrition Assistance Program: Examining the Evidence to Define Benefit Adequacy.* The National Academies Press, 2013.

[30] U.S. Census Bureau. URL: https://www.census.gov.

[31] U.S. Census Bureau. *2010 Census Urban and Rural Classifcation and Urban Area Criteria.*

[32] U.S. Census Bureau. *Current Population Survey.* URL: https://www.census.gov/programs-surveys/cps.html.

[33] U.S. Census Bureau. *State Area Measurements and Internal Point Coordinates.* URL: https://www.census.gov/geographies.html.

[34] U.S. Census Bureau. Table 6: People Below 125 Percent of Poverty Level and the Near Poor; Table 9: Poverty of People, by Region; Table 22: Number and Percent of People Below 50 Percent of Poverty Level. *Historical Poverty Tables: People and Families.*

[35] U.S. Census Bureau. *TIGER/Line® Shapefiles.* URL: https://www.census.gov/geo.

[36] U.S. Census Bureau. *Fifteenth Census of the United States: 1930, Population, Volume II, General Report, Statistics by Subject,* 1933.

[37] U.S. Census Bureau. Table HINC-01: Selected Characteristics of Households, by Total Money Income. *Current Population Survey, Annual Social and Economic Supplement,* 2006, 2011, and 2017.

[38] U.S. Census Bureau. Poverty and Median Household Income Estimates–Counties, States, and National. *Small Area Income and Poverty Estimates (SAIPE) Program,* 2013–2017.

[39] U.S. Census Bureau. Table DP03: Selected Economic Characteristics; Table DP04: Selected Housing Characteristics. *American Community Survey 5-Year Estimates,* 2013–2017.

[40] U.S. Census Bureau. Historical Table A-1: Educational Attainment in the United States. *Current Population Survey, Annual Social and Economic Supplement,* 2016.

[41] U.S. Census Bureau. Annual Estimates of the Resident Population: April 1, 2010 to July 1, 2018. *Population Estimates Program,* 2017.

[42] U.S. Census Bureau. Poverty Thresholds for 2017 by Size of Family and Number of Related Children Under 18 Years, 2017.

[43] U.S. Census Bureau. Table B01003: Total Population. *American Community Survey 1-Year Estimates and Population Estimates Program,* 2017.

[44] U.S. Census Bureau. Table B19083: Gini Index of Income Inequality by State. *American Community Survey 1-Year Estimates,* 2017.

[45] U.S. Census Bureau. Table S1901: Income in the Past 12 Months (In 2017 Inflation-Adjusted Dollars). *American Community Survey 1-Year Estimates,* 2017.

[46] W.A. Chance. A note on the origins of index numbers. *The Review of Economics and Statistics,* 48(1):108–110, 1966.

[47] L.T. Chang. *Factory Girls: From Village to City in a Changing China.* Spiegel & Grau, 2008.

[48] C.F. Citro and R.T. Michaels, editors. *Measuring Poverty: A New Approach.* The National Academies Press, 1995.

[49] E. Cofer, E. Grossman, and F. Clark. *Family Food Plans and Food Costs, Home Economics Research Report No. 20.* U.S. Department of Agriculture, 1962.

[50] U.S. Congress. *An Act Making appropriations for the Department of Agriculture for the fiscal year ending June thirtieth, eighteen hundred and ninety-five.* Fifty-third Congress, Session II, Ch. 238, August 8, 1894.

[51] U.S. Congress. *An Act Supplementary to the Acts in Relation to Immigration*. Forty-third Congress, Session II, Ch. 141, March 3, 1875.

[52] U.S. Congress. *An Act To Execute Certain Treaty Stipulations Relating to Chinese*. Forty-seventh Congress, Session I, Ch. 126, May 6, 1882.

[53] U.S. Congress, Office of Technology Assessment. *An Assessment of the United States Food and Agricultural Research System*, 1981.

[54] A. Deaton. *The Great Escape: Health, Wealth, and the Origins of Inequality*. Princeton University Press, 2013.

[55] U.S. Department of Agriculture. *Food Consumption of Households in the United States*. Household Food Consumption Survey 1955, Report No. 1, December 1956.

[56] U.S. Department of Housing and Urban Development. *HUD USPS ZIP Code Crosswalk Files*. URL: https://www.huduser.gov.

[57] U.S. Department of Housing and Urban Development. Table C-01-AH-M: General Housing Data for San Diego-Carlsbad-San Marcos AHS Area in 2011. *American Housing Survey*, 2011.

[58] U.S. Department of the Interior. *U.S. Geological Survey–Earthquake Hazards Program*. URL: https://earthquake.usgs.gov/.

[59] U.S. Department of the Interior, Census Office. *Report on Population of the United States at the Eleventh Census: 1890, Vol. 1, Part II*, 1897.

[60] M. Desmond. *Evicted: Poverty and Profit in the American City*. The Crown Publishing Group, 2016.

[61] C. Dickens. *Oliver Twist*. Penguin Classics, reissue edition 2003.

[62] W.E. Diewert and A.O. Nakamura, editors. *Essays in Index Number Theory, Volume 1*. Elsevier Science Publishers B.V., 1993.

[63] K. Dill. Report: CEOs earn 331 times as much as average workers, 774 times as much as minimum wage earners. *Forbes*, April 15, 2014.

[64] N. Eberstadt, R. Nunn, D.W. Schanzenbach, and M.R. Strain. *"In order that they might rest their arguments on facts": The vital role of government-collected data*. The Hamilton Project at the Brookings Institution and the American Enterprise Institute, March 2017.

[65] B. Ehrenreich. *Nickel and Dimed: On (Not) Getting By in America*. Picador, 2011.

[66] Encyclopædia Britannica, Inc. *Entry on the "Personal Computer."* URL: https://www.britannica.com/technology/personal-computer.

[67] V. Eubanks. *Automating Inequality: How High-Tech Tools Profile, Police, and Punish the Poor*. St. Martin's Press, 2018.

[68] European Communities. *The EEC Begins War on Want in the Community*. European Communities Commission Press Release ISEC/85/75, November 28, 1975.

[69] Eurostat. *People at risk of poverty or social exclusion*. URL: https://ec.europa.eu/eurostat/.

[70] U.S. Federal Housing Finance Agency. *House Price Index*. URL: https://www.fhfa.gov.

[71] J. Flanigan. Unlike stocks, home prices rarely collapse. *Los Angeles Times*, August 28, 1988.

[72] W. Fleetwood. *Chronicon Preciosum: Or, an Account of English Money, the Price of Corn, and Other Commodities, for the Last 600 Years. In a Letter to a Student in the University of Oxford.* Charles Harper, 1707.

[73] L. Fox. The supplemental poverty measure: 2017 Technical report, U.S. Census Bureau, September 2018.

[74] T.I. Garner. Supplemental Poverty Measure thresholds: Laying the foundation. *Paper Prepared for Allied Social Science Associations Annual Meetings, Denver*, 2010.

[75] J.L. Gastwirth. The estimation of the Lorenz curve and Gini index. *The Review of Economics and Statistics*, 54(3):306–316, 1972.

[76] J.G. Gauthier. *Measuring America: The Decennial Censuses from 1790 to 2000.* U.S. Census Bureau, September 2002.

[77] G.M. Giorgi and S. Gubbiotti. Celebrating the memory of Corrado Gini: A personality out of the ordinary. *International Statistical Review*, 85(2):325–339, 2017.

[78] J.P. Goldberg and W.T. Moye. *The First Hundred Years of the Bureau of Labor Statistics.* U.S. Bureau of Labor Statistics, Bulletin 2235, September 1985.

[79] U.S. Government Accountability Office. High-Risk Series: Progress on Many High-Risk Areas, While Substantial Efforts Needed on Others. *GAO-17-317*, February 2017.

[80] T. Grondine. After 50+ years, Red Delicious falls to #2 as most grown U.S. apple, Gala takes #1 spot. *U.S. Apple Association*, August 23, 2018.

[81] T. Harford. Tim Harford's guide to statistics in a misleading age. *Financial Times*, February 8, 2018.

[82] P. Hodgson. Top CEOs make more than 300 times the average worker. *Fortune*, June 22, 2015.

[83] P. Holley. An artist hated the 'Fearless Girl' statue—so he put this at her feet. *The Washington Post*, May 30, 2017.

[84] C.L. Hunt. Food for young children. *U.S. Department of Agriculture, Farmers' Bulletin No. 717*, March 4, 1916.

[85] ILO/IMF/OECD/UNECE/Eurostat/The World Bank. *Consumer Price Index Manual: Theory and Practice.* International Labour Office, 2004.

[86] International Labour Organization, ISOSTAT (used with permission). URL: https://www.ilo.org.

[87] L.B. Johnson. *Annual Message to the Congress on the State of the Union*, January 8, 1964.

[88] Z. Karabell. *The Leading Indicators: A Short History of the Numbers That Rule Our World.* Simon & Schuster Paperbacks, 2014.

[89] J.M. Keynes. Economic possibilities for our grandchildren (1930). In *Essays in Persuasion*, pages 358–373. Harcourt, Brace & Company, 1931.

[90] C. Kleiber and S. Kotz. *Statistical Size Distributions in Economics and Actuarial Sciences.* John Wiley & Sons, Inc., 2003.

[91] N.F. Koehn. Great Men, great pay? Why CEO compensation is sky high. *The Washington Post*, June 12, 2014.

[92] A. LaFrance. A history of technology, via the Consumer Price Index. *The Atlantic*, April 5, 2016.

[93] D.F. Larcker, N.E. Donatiello, and B. Tayan. *Americans and CEO Pay: 2016 Public Perception Survey on CEO Compensation*. CGRI Survey Series. Corporate Governance Research Initiative, Stanford Rock Center for Corporate Governance, February 2016 (used with permission).

[94] C. LeBovit, E. Cofer, J. Murray, and F. Clark. *Dietary Evaluation of Food Used in Households in the United States, Household Food Consumption Survey 1955, Report No. 16.* U.S. Department of Agriculture, 1961.

[95] R. Lightner and T. Francis. Highest paid CEOs in America: Compensation for the chief executives of companies listed in the S&P 500 index. *The Wall Street Journal*, Accessed March 17, 2017.

[96] London School of Economics. *Charles Booth's London: Poverty Maps and Police Notebooks, 1886–1903*. URL: https://booth.lse.ac.uk.

[97] M.O. Lorenz. Methods of measuring the concentration of wealth. *Publications of the American Statistical Association*, 9(70):209–219, 1905.

[98] J. Madison. Census of the Union. In *Annals of Congress, House of Representatives, 1st Congress, 2nd Session*, February 2, 1790.

[99] M.E. Magnello. Karl Pearson's Gresham Lectures: W.F.R. Weldon, speciation and the origins of Pearsonian statistics. *The British Journal for the History of Science*, 29(1):43–63, 1996.

[100] R.D. McFadden. SoHo gift to Wall St.: A 3 1/2-ton bronze bull. *The New York Times*, December 16, 1989.

[101] A. Melin and J.S. Diamond. How companies justify big pay raises for CEOs. *Bloomberg*, June 4, 2015.

[102] UK Ministry of Housing, Communities & Local Government. *English Indices of Deprivation 2015*.

[103] MIT Sloane School of Management and Harvard Business School. *The Billion Prices Project*. URL: http://www.thebillionpricesproject.com/.

[104] N. Mohamud. Mana Musa: The richest man who ever lived. *BBC.com*, March 10, 2019.

[105] J.Z. Muller. *The Tyranny of Metrics*. Princeton University Press, 2018.

[106] H.B. Myers and J.N. Webb. Another census of unemployment? *American Journal of Sociology*, 42(4):521–533, 1937.

[107] C.H. Nagaraja, L.D. Brown, and L.H. Zhao. An autoregressive approach to house price modeling. *Annals of Applied Statistics*, 5(1):124–149, 2011.

[108] National Bureau of Economic Research. *U.S. Business Cycle Expansions and Contractions*. URL: https://www.nber.org/cycles.html.

[109] National Council of the Churches of Christ in the United States of America. *New Revised Standard Version Bible*, 1989. URL: http://www.biblegateway.com.

[110] The National Nutrition Conference. *Public Health Reports*, 56(24):1233–1255, 1941.

[111] National Planning Commission. *Namibia Index of Multiple Deprivation.* Republic of Namibia, 2015.

[112] M. Noble, H. Barnes, G. Wright, D. McLennan, D. Avenell, A. Whitworth, and B. Roberts. *The South African Index of Multiple Deprivation 2001 at Datazone Level.* Pretoria, Department of Social Development, 2009.

[113] A. O'Connor. *Poverty Knowledge: Social Science, Social Policy, and the Poor in Twentieth-Century U.S. History.* Princeton University Press, 2001.

[114] Office of Management and Budget. *Metropolitan and Micropolitan.* URL: https://www.census.gov/programs-surveys/metro-micro/about.html.

[115] Office of Management and Budget. *Statistical Policy Directive No. 14.* May 1978.

[116] Office of Management and Budget. Request for comment on the consumer inflation measures produced by federal statistical agencies. *Federal Register,* 84(88), May 7, 2019.

[117] U.S. Office of the Secretary of State. *Return of the Whole Number of Persons Within the Several Districts of the United States According to, "An Act Providing for the Enumeration of the Inhabitants of the United States,"* 1793.

[118] OnThisDay.com. *Historical Events in 1963.*

[119] M. Orshansky. How poverty is measured. *Monthly Labor Review,* 92:37–41, February 1969.

[120] M. Orshansky. Counting the poor: Another look at the poverty profile. *Social Security Bulletin,* pages 3–13, January 1965.

[121] B.W. Patch. Expansion of the food-stamp plan. *Editorial Research Reports, CQ Press,* Vol. 1, 1940.

[122] J. Pepitone. Hundreds of protesters descend to 'Occupy Wall Street.' *CNN Money,* September 17, 2011.

[123] M.J. Perry. New BLS data show that for all 'chief executives,' the 'average CEO-to-average worker pay ratio' is less than 5-to-1. *American Enterprise Institute,* March 31, 2016 (used with permission).

[124] K. Phillips. Numbers racket: Why the economy is worse than we know. *Harper's Magazine,* pages 43–47, May 2008.

[125] T. Piketty and A. Goldhammer (translator). *Capital in the Twenty-First Century.* Belknap Press of Harvard University Press, 2014.

[126] T. Piketty and A. Goldhammer (translator). *The Economics of Inequality.* Belknap Press of Harvard University Press, 2015.

[127] S.B. Reed. One hundred years of price change: The Consumer Price Index and the American inflation experience. *Monthly Labor Review,* April 2014.

[128] T. Renwick. Geographic adjustments of Supplemental Poverty Measure thresholds: Using the American Community Survey five-year data on housing costs. *U.S. Census Bureau,* SEHSD Working Paper Number 2011-21, 2011.

[129] D. Rippy. The first hundred years of the Consumer Price Index: A methodological and political history. *Monthly Labor Review,* April 2014.

[130] F.D. Roosevelt. Fireside Chat on the Unemployment Census. In *Speeches of President Franklin D. Roosevelt, 1933-1945.* November 14, 1937.

[131] T. Rose. *The End of Average: How We Succeed in a World That Values Sameness.* HarperOne, 2016.

[132] A.M. Ross. Living with symbols. *The American Statistician*, 20(3):15–18, 1966.

[133] B.S. Rowntree. *Poverty: A Study of Town Life.* Macmillan and Co., Limited, 1901.

[134] B.S. Rowntree. *The Human Needs of Labour.* Thomas Nelson and Sons, Ltd., 1918.

[135] C. Sandburg. Chicago. *Poetry*, Vol. III, No. VI, 1914.

[136] M.J. Sandel. *What Money Can't Buy: The Moral Limits of Markets.* Farrar, Straus and Giroux, 2013.

[137] Securities and Exchange Commission. *SEC Adopts Rule for Pay Ratio Disclosure.* August 5, 2015. URL: https://www.sec.gov/news/pressrelease/2015-160.html.

[138] A. Sen. Poor, relatively speaking. *Oxford Economic Papers, New Series*, 35(2):153–169, 1983.

[139] R.J. Shiller. *Irrational Exuberance: Revised and Expanded Third Edition.* Princeton University Press, 2015.

[140] A. Shorrocks, J. Davies, and R. Lluberas. *Global Wealth Report 2018.* Credit Suisse Research Institute, October 2018 (used with permission).

[141] G. Skinner, J. Stannard, and O. Lohoar Self. *Perils of Perception 2018.* Ipsos MORI, 2018.

[142] L. Soth. Henry Wallace and the farm crisis of the 1920s and 1930s. *The Annals of Iowa*, 47(2):195–214, 1983.

[143] L. Stack. 'Fearless Girl' statue to stay in financial district (for now). *The New York Times*, March 27, 2017.

[144] Standard and Poor's Financial Services LLC. *S&P CoreLogic Case–Shiller Home Price Indices* (used with permission). URL: https://us.spindices.com/.

[145] T.A. Stapleford. *The Cost of Living in America: A Political History of Economic Statistics, 1880–2000.* Cambridge University Press, 2009.

[146] H.K. Stiebeling. *Are We Well Fed? A Report on the Diets of Families in the United States.* U.S. Department of Agriculture, Miscellaneous Publication No. 430, 1941.

[147] J.E. Stiglitz. *The Great Divide: Unequal Societies and What We Can Do About Them.* W.W. Norton & Company, Inc., 2015.

[148] J.E. Stiglitz and L.J. Bilmes. The 1 percent's problem. *Vanity Fair*, May 31, 2012.

[149] J. Suzman. *Affluence Without Abundance: The Disappearing World of the Bushmen.* Bloomsbury USA, 2017.

[150] E.B. Tylor. Physique sociale, ou essai sur le développement des facultés de l'homme anthropométrie, ou misure des différentes facultés de l'homme. *Nature*, 5:358–363, 1872.

[151] Valuation Technology Inc. (used with permission). URL: http://valuationtechnology.com.

[152] J.D. Vance. *Hillbilly Elegy: A Memoir of a Family and Culture in Crisis.* HarperCollins Publishers, 2016.

[153] T. Vigen. *Spurious Correlations.* URL: https://www.tylervigen.com/spurious-correlations.

[154] A. Walker, D. Gordon, R. Levitas, P. Phillimore, C. Phillipson, M.E. Salomon, and N. Yeates, editors. *The Peter Townsend Reader.* Policy Press, 2010.

[155] War Food Administration, Nutrition and Food Conservation Branch. *National Wartime Nutrition Guide, NFC-4.* U.S. Department of Agriculture, July 1943.

[156] J.N. Webb. Concepts used in unemployment surveys. *Journal of the American Statistical Association,* 34(205):49–59, 1939.

[157] F.M. Williams. Bureau of Labor Statistics Cost-of-Living Index in wartime. *Monthly Labor Review,* 57:82–100, July 1943.

[158] K.C.M. Wilson, S. Taylor, J.R.M. Copeland, R. Chen, and C.F.M. McCracken. Socio-economic deprivation and the prevalence and prediction of depression in older community residents: The MRC-ALPHA study. *The British Journal of Psychiatry,* 175:549–553, 1999.

[159] World Bank. GINI Index (World Bank Estimate). URL: http://data.worldbank.org/indicator.

[160] World Bank. *Poverty & Equity Data Portal.* URL: http://povertydata.worldbank.org/poverty/home/.

[161] World Inequality Database. URL: https://wid.world/.

[162] T. Worstall. The average CEO makes four times the average worker. *Forbes,* May 2, 2015.

[163] C.D. Wright and W.O. Hunt. The History and Growth of the United States Census: Prepared for the Senate Committee on the Census. In *56th Congress, 1st Session, Document No. 194,* February 24, 1900.

[164] Zillow Group. *Zillow Home Value Index.* URL: https://www.zillow.com.

[165] H. Zinn. *A People's History of the United States.* Harper Perennial Model Classics, 2015 edition.

Index

American Enterprise Institute (AEI), 26–29, 153
American Federation of Labor and Congress of Industrial Organizations (AFL–CIO), 26–28
American Statistical Association, 11
Atwater, William O., 97, 100, 108
average, *see also* mean

bar graph, **40**, **62**, *155*
Billion Prices Project, 96
Black Report, 127
Booth, Charles, 107, 108, 118, 122, 128, **128**, 129, 130, 132, 146
Boskin, Michael, 83
Bowley, Arthur Lyon, 122
Brookings Institution, 153
Bureau of Economic Analysis (BEA), 72, 93, 104
Personal Consumption Expenditure Index (PCE), 72, 77, 78
Bureau of Labor Statistics (BLS), 4, 5, 11, 12, **14**, 22, 27, **73**, **81**, **86**, **89**, **92**, 71–96, 108, 112, **121**, *155*
Commodities and Services (C&S) sample, 91, 93, 95

Consumer Expenditure (CE) Survey, 85, 87, 88, 90, 93–95, 112, **114, 115, 119**, *156*
Consumer Price Index (CPI), **81**, **86**, **89**, **92**, 71–96
CPI Housing Survey, 93
Current Employment Statistics (CES) program, 12, 22
Telephone Point of Purchase Survey (TPOPS), 90

Carli, Gian Rinaldo, 74
Carter, Jimmy, 84
Census Bureau, 12, 39, 53, **54**, 104, 105, 112, **113**, 114, **121, 122**, 124, 125, 152, *155*
American Community Survey (ACS), **47**, 106, 116, **117**, 132, **135, 137**, 138, **139, 140, 142, 145**, *155*
American Housing Survey (AHS), 53, **55**, 93, *155*
Current Population Survey (CPS), 8, **9**, 12, 13, **15**, 16, **17, 20**, 22, 42, **43**, 104, 105, **105**, 124, *157*

decennial census, 6, 10, 23, **144, 145,** *157*
Population Estimates Program (PEP), *158*
Small Area Income and Poverty Estimates (SAIPE) program, 106, 114, 124, 137, **139, 140, 142,** *160*
Supplemental Poverty Measure (SPM), 116, 118–120, **121,** 122, **122,** 124, 125
centering, 133, 134
confidence interval, **122,** 123, 124, *156*
Core Based Statistical Area (CBSA), 53, **54**
correlation, 129, 130, **131,** 137, 141, 143, 146, *156*
cost of living, 77, 82, 83, 93–96
Credit Suisse Research Institute, 31, 32

Deaton, Angus, 149
Department of Agriculture (USDA), 97, 99, **99,** 100, 101, 103, 106, 124
deprivation, 3, 126–150
Dodd–Frank Wall Street Reform and Consumer Protection Act, 29, 30

Federal Housing and Finance Agency (FHFA), 52, 67, **68**
Federal Reserve Bank, 72, 84, 93
Fisher's ideal index, 76, 77, 80, 94
Fleetwood, William, 74
Ford, Gerald, 83

geometric mean, 76, 77, 94, *157*
Gini coefficient, 38–47
Gini, Corrado, 42

Harding, Warren G., 11
histogram, **43, 47, 62, 64, 66,** 133, 143, **144,** *157*
Hoover, Herbert, 5, 11, 82
house price index, 51–70, 72, 80, 90

Index of Multiple Deprivation, 127, 131, 147
inequality, 3, 24–49, 58
inflation, 1, 4, 59, 62, 69–96, 98, 104, 112, 119, 124
International Labour Organization (ILO), 19, **21**
Ipsos Group S.A., 151

Johnson, Lyndon B., 103, 107, 109, 125

Keynes, John Maynard, 18

labor force participation rate, 6–10
Laspeyres index, 76, 77, 80, 83, 94, 95
Lincoln, Abraham, 99
logarithm, 63, 64, **64,** 133
Lorenz curve, 38–47
Lorenz, Max Otto, vii, 39, 42
Lowe, Joseph, 75
Lubin, Isador, 11

Madison, James, 151
mean, 51, 52, **52, 57,** 55–60, 63, 65, **73,** 72–78, 89, 130–136, *157*
median, 29, 30, **52, 57,** 55–59, 61, **62,** 65, 67, 69, *157*

Meeker, Royal, 78

National Bureau of Economic Research (NBER), **9**, **15**, **17**, **20**, **21**, **34**, **37**, **57**, **60**, **62**, **68**, **81**, **105**, *158*
Nixon, Richard, 83, 91

Obama, Barack, 29, 116
Occupy Wall Street, 25, 31
Office of Management and Budget (OMB), 53, 111
official statistic, 1, 3, 19, 111, 151, 153, *158*
Orshansky, Mollie, 102–104, 107–112, 118, 124
outlier, 30, 58, 63, **64**, 134, **135**, 136, 146, *158*

Paasche index, 76, 77, 94
Pearson, Karl, 42
percent change, 72, 80, **81**, 82, **92**, 95, *158*
percentile, 30–45, 138, **139**, **140**, 141, 147, *158*
Perkins, Frances, 11, 82, 83
Pigou–Dalton principle, 45, 46
Piketty, Thomas, 48, *161*
population, *158*
poverty, 2, 3, 70, 97–150
price relative, 58, 72, **73**, 74, 75, 78, *158*

quantile, *see also* percentile
Quetelet, Adolphe, 51, 52

ratio statistic, 6, *158*
regression, 63, 65
repeat sales, **52**, **66**, **67**, **68**, 61–69
robust, 30, *159*

Roosevelt, Franklin D., 5, 11, 12, 23, 82, 83, 101, 106
Rowntree, Benjamin Seebohm, 108, 118, 122
Royal Statistical Society, **128**

sample, *159*
sampling frame, *159*
scatterplot, **128**, 129, **131**, 141, **142**, 143, **145**, 146, *159*
seasonality, seasonal adjustment, 8, **9**, 10, 15, 16, 59, **60**, 69, 80, 87, 91, 93, *159*
Sen, Amartya, 98, 109
Shiller, Robert J., 65, 67, 69
skew, 63, **64**, 65, *159*
Smith, Adam, 109
Standard & Poor's Financial Services LLC, 52, 67, **68**
standard deviation, 130–136, *160*
standardization, 134, 136, *160*
standarization, **135**
statistic, *160*
Stewart, Ethelbert, 11
Stigler, George, 83, 93, 94

Törnqvist index, 94
time series, 8, **9**, 15, **15**, **17**, **20**, **21**, **34**, **37**, **57**, **60**, **62**, **68**, **73**, **81**, **86**, **92**, *160*
Townsend Material Deprivation Index, 130–149
Trump, Donald J., 29, 104, 112

unemployment, 1, 4–23, 27, 36, 71, 82, 101, 103, 104, 107, 110, 124, 151

Valuation Technology Inc., **57,
60**, **62**, 64, **66**, **67**
Vaughan, Rice, 74

Wallace, Henry A., 106
Washington, George, *157*
Wilson, Woodrow, 100
Works Progress Administration
(WPA), 12, 18
World Bank, 46, 97, 98, 109
World Inequality Database
(WID.world), **34**, **36**,
37, **40**, *161*

Zillow Group, 52, 67, **68**